P9-BEE-411

CORE ENVY

CORE ENVY

A 3-STEP GUIDE TO A STRONG, SEXY CORE

ALLISON WESTFAHL

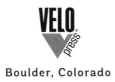

Boulder, Colorado

Copyright © 2016 by Allison Westfahl

All rights reserved. Printed in the United States of America.

No part of this book may be reproduced, stored in a retrieval system, or transmitted, in any form or by any means, electronic or photocopy or otherwise, without the prior written permission of the publisher except in the case of brief quotations within critical articles and reviews.

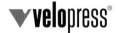

3002 Sterling Circle, Suite 100
Boulder, Colorado 80301-2338 USA
(303) 440-0601 · Fax (303) 444-6788 · E-mail velopress@competitorgroup.com

Distributed in the United States and Canada by Ingram Publisher Services

A Cataloging-in-Publication record for this book is available from the Library of Congress.
ISBN 978-1-937715-34-2

For information on purchasing VeloPress books,
please call (800) 811-4210, ext. 2138, or visit www.velopress.com.

This paper meets the requirements of ANSI/NISO Z39.48-1992 (Permanence of Paper).

Cover and interior design by Katie Jennings Design
Cover photograph by Matt Hawthorne
Interior and back cover photographs by Julia Vandenoever
Photo-shoot location courtesy of Pura Vida Fitness & Spa

16   17   18 / 10   9   8   7   6   5   4   3   2

CONTENTS

The Core Envy Workout Plan

ACKNOWLEDGMENTS

When I sat down with the team at VeloPress in the spring of 2014 to discuss this project, I had no idea what a labor of love it would turn out to be. Throughout the entire process, I have received incredible support from countless people:

Renee Jardine, editor extraordinaire. Her attention to detail is truly tireless, as is her creative vision.

The entire team at VeloPress, especially Vicki Hopewell, Connie Oehring, Dave Trendler, and Julia Vandenoever.

My incredible families. I couldn't have asked for a better family to have been born into (the Westfahls) or married into (the Wagners).

All of the women who motivated and inspired me to create this plan over the years. Go get that enviable core!

My dog, Muppet. Sometimes a fuzzy snuggle and a friendly paw are all I need to find motivation.

And most of all, my husband, Brian, whose encouragement and unconditional support have given me the confidence to take on challenges I thought were impossible. It's a true gift to spend every day with your best friend and partner in crime.

INTRODUCTION

When I take on new clients, I have them fill out a questionnaire to help me better understand their fitness goals. Clients are asked to rank potential areas of focus in order of importance—core strength, weight loss, muscle toning, injury rehab, better energy, etc. The top three are almost always the same, especially when it comes to my female clients: Core strength is the primary goal, followed by weight loss and toning.

It's not surprising that most women are looking to improve their core; after all, the term "core strength" has become practically synonymous with "fitness" in the past decade. We've all been told that a stronger core is absolutely essential to good health, fewer aches and pains, and most importantly a better physique. There is certainly no shame in wanting a more defined midsection. After all, isn't that what we're all saying when we profess to wanting greater core strength?

As women, we are presented with an overwhelming number of products, supplements, and workouts that promise a tighter tummy and perfect six-pack abs. The irony about that flashy six-pack is that it does not in any way imply that you have functional core strength, yet it continues to be the hallmark of a fit, sexy body. The pursuit of goddesslike abs is the reason we are willing to engage in self-inflicted torture—hundreds of crunches, a cycle of diets and cleanses, and a litany of unregulated supplements that claim to burn belly fat in mere minutes. In our desperation to find a solution to the flabby abby, we can be easily swayed by perfectly sculpted models, most of whom did not get chiseled abs by using the product they are promoting. The problem is that most of these efforts deliver short-lived results, if any at all, and leave us utterly frustrated. How can we keep our waistlines from expanding without starving ourselves or devoting hours a day to grueling workouts? Why isn't there a solution that is both effective and sustainable? These are questions that I hear from my clients on a daily basis, and this is why I developed the Core Envy program: to give you a strong, sexy core that is functional and looks great.

You might look at me and assume that I can't empathize with your fitness struggle, but let me assure you that I've run into many of the same dead ends you have in my attempts to control my waistline. Growing up, I was never categorized as overweight, but I certainly was never referred to as "thin." In fact, the term that was most often used to describe me was "stocky," which basically meant I was short and thick. I never paid attention to food or calories because I was an athlete and thought I needed the fuel for performance.

When I got to college I was confronted with a frightening reality—no more team sports and an unlimited dessert bar in the dining hall. I was well aware of the "freshman 15," but I didn't think it would happen to me. I was putting in 30-minute sessions on the elliptical at the fitness center and walking to class—surely that had to burn lots of calories! By sophomore year I had managed to put on close to 20 pounds, which is pretty noticeable on a stocky 5-foot-2-inch frame. I clearly remember the day at the end of my sophomore year when I could no longer button my jeans. In a fit of panic I immediately started doing crunches, hoping that my waistline would magically shrink over the course of the next 100 repetitions. It didn't, but I continued to incorporate crunches into my exercise routine for more years than I like to acknowledge, convinced that if I abandoned this time-honored exercise routine, I would surely be tempting the muffin-top gods. It took a master's degree in exercise science, scores of scientific studies, and—most convincingly—personal experience to persuade me to ditch the crunches and turn to a more integrated approach in order to achieve an enviable core.

In this book, I'll share with you what I've learned about achieving and maintaining a strong, sexy core. I've done my research; vetted my approach with thousands of clients over the past 15 years; and landed on a program that is effective, is easy to follow, and won't leave you in a continued state of frustration and dismay. I can't promise you a flat stomach overnight, but if you have 8 weeks to devote to a program based on fact, not fad, you will see a significant change in your core.

WHAT YOU CAN EXPECT

This program is designed for real people with real time constraints, real jobs, real families, and a real desire to follow a program that isn't complicated. I'm not going to ask you to do hundreds of crunches, set aside two hours a day for workouts, or spend money on weird vegetables and supplements that aren't normally a part of your diet. My Core Envy program integrates three routines to build a strong, sexy core:

- Sculpting exercises to tighten and tone
- Cardio workouts to melt belly fat
- A diet makeover to help you reach your goals

Along the way, I'll explain the science behind the workouts, helping you feel confident that you're devoting your time to a program that is effective and efficient.

We live in an age of information overload. With so many promises of overnight results being thrown at you from all directions, you deserve to know the relevant facts about your health and your body. I'm not going to sugarcoat the process or make outlandish claims that you can have a better body with "5 easy moves." Getting fit and staying fit takes time and dedication, but the experience doesn't have to be a miserable one. My Core Envy program can be tailored to fit your lifestyle and your current level of fitness. I'll show you how to choose the most powerful forms of sculpting, cardio, and nutrition to transform your core.

SETTING YOURSELF UP FOR SUCCESS

Maybe this is your first fitness book, or maybe it's your fiftieth. Either way, I want it to be your last. The Core Envy program can help you achieve your goals, but in order to do that you need to set yourself up for success. There are a few things that are essential to maximizing your results—if you can focus on these three things, you will greatly increase your chances of sticking to this program and finally achieving the core you want.

1. Today is the perfect day to start. Yes, I know that you have the company holiday party next week and that your best friend's birthday is the following Tuesday, but guess what? Life is always happening, and there will always be the perfect excuse for why you can't start living a healthy lifestyle right now. The biggest disservice that we do ourselves is expecting 100 percent perfection 100 percent of the time and then deciding that anything less is failure. Start the Core Envy program today, then go to that holiday party next week and do the best you can. If you make food choices that you're unhappy with, don't throw in the towel and decide that all the work you did the week before was worthless. Health is the cumulative effect of choices you make over time. I'm guessing it took you more than a week to gain the extra weight that you're carrying around your tummy, so don't expect it to go away in a week. Make a commitment to yourself today. And the next day, and the next ...

2. Schedule your entire day around your workout. Study after study shows that people who work out first thing in the morning are exponentially more likely to work out regularly. Why? Because emergencies at work or home are much more common at 6 p.m. than at 6 a.m. Set your alarm and get your workout done before the rest of the day takes over. If the morning hours just aren't an option, then put your workout in your calendar and make sure that everyone around you knows that block of time is non-negotiable. If you are like me, you might have to get a little creative in blocking out your time. Because many of my personal training clients switch their day and time from week to week, I've learned that I must block off time in my calendar for my own workouts or else I run the risk of scheduling too many clients and not leaving any breaks for myself. I used to write "workout" in my calendar, but then I had one too many clients look over my shoulder and ask if I could move my workout because it was the only time that worked for her to come in. After sacrificing my own workouts numerous times, I started writing "Dana" on my schedule for my personal workout. I even had one client comment, "Dana seems super dedicated—she comes in almost every day!" I

just smiled and said, "Yes, and she's seeing great results!"

3. Surround yourself with support. Don't try to go through this journey on your own. Let your family, friends, and colleagues know that you're making a commitment to living healthier and ask them to help keep you accountable. The most important people to have on board are the people with whom you live because they have the ability to encourage or sabotage your progress with the foods they bring into the house. It's very difficult to stay true to your nutrition plan when you're surrounded by chocolate-chip cookies and potato chips! Maybe the people in your life need a little encouragement in this area as well, so recruit your friends to do the Core Envy program with you.

If you find yourself struggling, want to share your journey, or need further information about the workouts and nutrition plan, please visit the Core Envy web site at www.coreenvybook.com.

3 steps to an
ENVIABLE CORE

Step 1: THE NEW RULES of
SCULPTING

LEFT TO OUR OWN DEVICES, most of us would begin a regimen of abdominal crunches to create an enviable core. It seems like the obvious and logical strategy. After all, if you want to improve upon something, you should do more of that thing. To improve your tennis serve, you practice serving; to improve your golf swing, you practice golfing; and so on. So the fastest road to a great-looking core is to dedicate more time to working your abs. A typical visit to the gym might include 30 minutes on the elliptical, 10 minutes of crunches, and a protein shake in the car. Sound like a familiar workout? If you've been following a program similar to this for months (maybe years?) and seen little to no change in your body, you're not alone. We've been programmed to think that crunches are the fastest path to a flat belly.

Our cultural obsession with crunches has deep roots, which I will attempt to extract throughout the course of this book. It's difficult to turn away from traditional, time-honored practices, mainly because they feel comfortable. Maybe you remember racing through a minute of crunches in PE to prove your fitness level. You've probably been to group fitness classes, all of which seemed to be some version of cardio exercise that ends with a series of crunches. Essentially, we have been trained to follow a workout template that consists of low-intensity cardio topped off with five variations of a traditional crunch. Despite all my education in exercise science, it took me years to break out of this workout doctrine because it was all I had ever known. Even though I wasn't seeing the results that I wanted, the female workout code of *elliptical + crunches = better body* was so embedded in my psyche that I felt deviating from it would amount to fitness heresy. I was scared. Sure, I could try something new and radical, but I was skeptical that the outcome would be any different. And even though my workout strategy wasn't working, I was really good at it.

I spent way too many years thinking that the length of my workout would be directly proportional to the results I would see. More is better! I kept adding more and more low-intensity cardio every time I wanted to drop a few pounds, more crunches if I wanted to tighten my tummy, and more diet sodas and sugar-free frozen yogurt to eat "healthier." Once I became a personal trainer and started coaching people, I noticed that my clients' workout history sounded eerily similar to my own. I quickly realized that we were getting it wrong—it was time to shed the traditional routine of cardio and crunches and do something radical. It was time to create a program that would deliver the results we were all looking for.

DON'T WASTE YOUR TIME WITH CRUNCHES

It might come as a shock that the Core Envy program does not include crunches. I've intentionally omitted them because they don't utilize a significant percentage of your core musculature. While it feels like you're working hard when you're 70 reps into a grueling round of 100 crunches, you are predominantly working a single muscle group—the rectus abdominis (rectus). In actuality, the true "core" of the body includes countless other muscles.

This brings up the issue of function versus vanity. Why wouldn't you want to focus your gym time on developing a rockin' rectus? Aren't those the beach muscles that look great with a spray tan? If a well-developed rectus is what turns heads, do we really need a well-rounded core routine that works all the other muscles? The short answer is that a high-functioning core leads to a better-looking core. Focusing on only a few core muscles can lead to poor posture (which makes your tummy stick out) and injuries (which will inhibit you from being able to work out). Build a solid foundation for your core with a well-rounded core routine, and you will

A high-functioning core leads to *a better-looking core.*

accomplish the dual goals of looking good while being strong and pain-free.

When I talk about the foundation for your core, I'm not referring just to the intricate musculature beneath your abs. Your glutes and hamstrings are also involved. These muscles are traditionally categorized as "lower-body" muscles, but they serve a dual function in helping to stabilize and move the pelvis, which makes them part of the core. In fact, any muscle that is attached to either the pelvis or the spine is technically part of the core. Add to the major muscle groups all of the smaller, deeper muscles in this area, and the count of how many muscles are in the human core eas-ily reaches into the hundreds. If your core strengthening routine is based solely on crunches, you're neglecting 95 percent of your core musculature.

When a large percentage of your core muscles is routinely ignored, it creates a scenario called *muscular imbalance* in which a muscle or group of muscles becomes tight and overactive, therefore causing a neighboring or opposing muscle to become weak and underactive. The imbalance is problematic because our muscles control our joints and bones, and when a certain muscle is doing too much work, it will start to pull the bones and joints it is attached to into uncomfortable positions.

AB EXERCISES *vs.* CORE EXERCISES

The terms "abs" and "core" are not synonymous, though they are often erroneously used interchangeably. The abdominal muscles consist of only four groups of muscles—the rectus abdominis, external obliques, internal obliques, and transverse abdominis—whereas the entire core consists of all the muscles (muscle groups) depicted in the figures on pages 10 and 11. You might have strong abs, but this does not mean your entire core is strong!

AB EXERCISES	CORE EXERCISES
Reverse crunch	Plank holds
Side crunch	Squats
Traditional crunch	Mountain climbers
Bicycle crunch	Bird dogs

CORE MUSCULATURE - FRONT

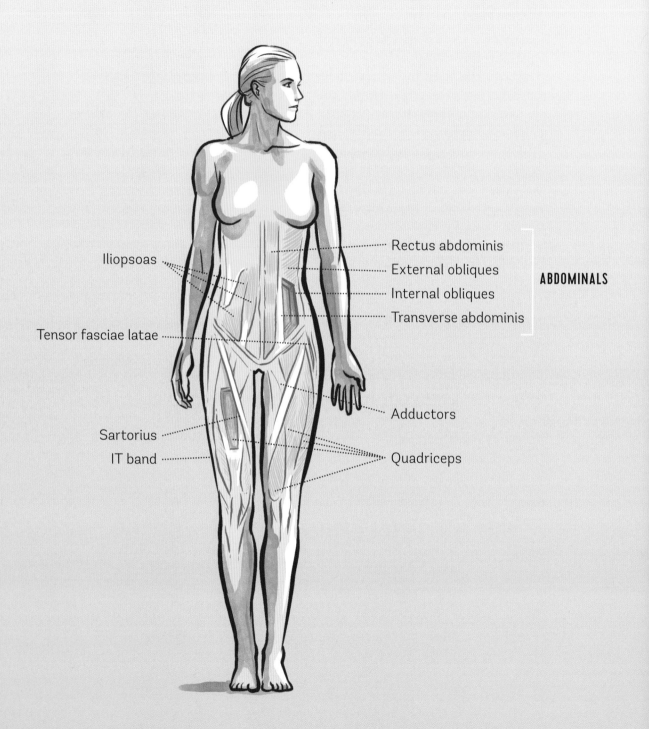

Iliopsoas

Tensor fasciae latae

Sartorius

IT band

Rectus abdominis

External obliques

Internal obliques

Transverse abdominis

ABDOMINALS

Adductors

Quadriceps

CORE MUSCULATURE - BACK

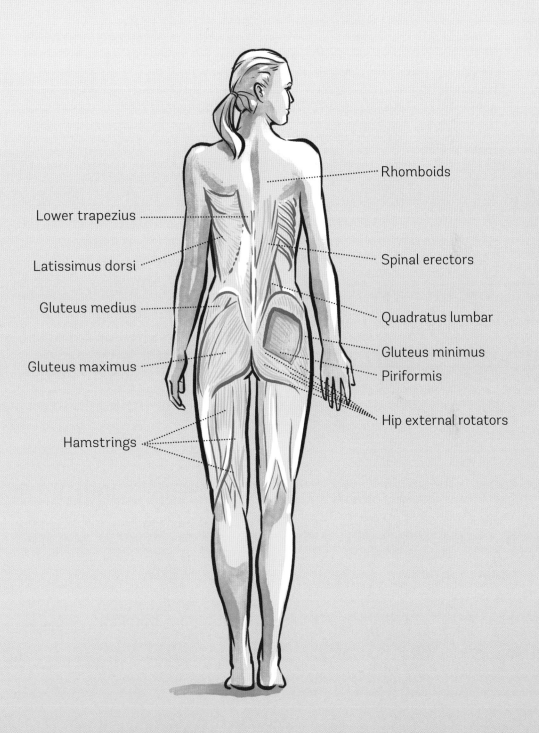

Rhomboids

Lower trapezius

Latissimus dorsi

Spinal erectors

Gluteus medius

Quadratus lumbar

Gluteus minimus

Gluteus maximus

Piriformis

Hip external rotators

Hamstrings

For example, when our friend the rectus abdominis becomes overactive, it pulls the rib cage and pelvis closer together. Repetitively bringing your rectus muscles into a contracted, or shortened, position results in poor posture and can ultimately place excessive pressure on the discs of the spine, causing pain and even long-term injury.

Most people have core musculature that is extremely imbalanced, primarily because we already do exercises that work on strengthening only the rectus. Such exercises are particularly problematic because we are already shortening our rectus all day while we sit in the car, sit at our desks, sit on the couch, or slouch while we walk. Simply stated, we don't need to work our rectus because is it already overworked and overactive.

Instead of doing exercises that shorten the rectus, we need to focus on exercises that recruit the deep core muscles. Scientific studies have actually proven that crunches and similar movements that involve trunk flexion do not activate the core muscles as effectively as do other exercises. In a recent study conducted at Auburn University, researchers tested the efficiency of popular core exercises through the use of electromyography.[1] By positioning electrodes on the skin over the muscles that are being tested, this technology measures the level of contraction found in those muscles. In order to establish a reference scale for the study, the standard crunch was assigned a value of 100. The exercises with values higher than 100 points showed greater muscular contraction than the standard crunch, and those under 100 had less. The results of the study clearly show why crunches are out, whereas moves such as the Pilates hundred and the isometric side bridge are in. The exercises that successfully recruit the deep abdominal muscles have two things in common: They require a high degree of stabilization, and they avoid trunk flexion. Additional movements that follow these guidelines include exercises such as the plank hold, the seated boat row, and windshield wipers. The Core Envy program uses variations of all of these movements and many more original movements I created to give you an enviable core that is also functional.

In addition to recruiting the deep core muscles, we need to recruit the big movers of the core, primarily the gluteals. You can't have an enviable core without having glutes that are strong and functional. I've had many a client make the argument that her butt is

That burn you feel in your abs during a crunch *does not mean that you're burning fat.*

CORE MUSCLES ENGAGED FOR SELECTED EXERCISES

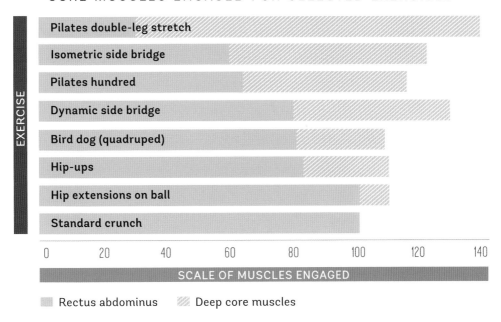

EXERCISE

- Pilates double-leg stretch
- Isometric side bridge
- Pilates hundred
- Dynamic side bridge
- Bird dog (quadruped)
- Hip-ups
- Hip extensions on ball
- Standard crunch

0   20   40   60   80   100   120   140

SCALE OF MUSCLES ENGAGED

▨ Rectus abdominus   ▨ Deep core muscles

* All exercises have been compared to standard crunch as baseline.

already big, so it must be strong. Well, we've all heard the adage, but in this case it's true: Size doesn't matter. It's entirely possible (and very common) to have glutes that take up a lot of real estate but aren't actually working. If you want to find out whether or not your glutes are showing up for the job, try the test in the sidebar on page 14. When the glutes are shut off and not firing correctly, the body will rely on other muscles to step in and do the job. Often the muscles that take over for the glutes are smaller (for example, the muscles of the low back) and less efficient. Over time, these muscles will become excessively taxed and will end up causing pain and injury.

BURN CALORIES WITH CARDIO, NOT CORE WORK

The term "burn" has been associated with exercise for a long time: Feel the burn, burn away fat, calorie burn, burning muscles…the list goes on and on. We all want to feel that the exercises we are doing are effective and worthwhile, and that burning sensation we get while doing a specific movement helps us feel that we are working hard, burning lots of calories, and therefore tightening the muscles that are burning. But what exactly is that burning sensation, and is it really a barometer for the effectiveness of a workout?

Are your GLUTES FIRING?

To test the firing capability of your glutes, perform this simple exercise. Lie on your back with your knees bent and your feet on the ground 8 to 10 inches from your glutes. Lift one leg off the floor. Pressing through the opposite heel, lift your hips as high off the ground as possible. You should feel this movement primarily in the glute of the leg pressing into the floor. Complete 15 repetitions, then switch to the other leg.

If you feel the movement in your glutes, then your posterior is functioning properly. If you feel it in your hamstrings and low back, then you need to focus on glute activation and strengthening exercises. Turn to page 191 to find a "Booty Bonus" series that will do just that.

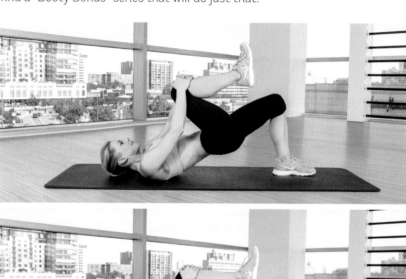

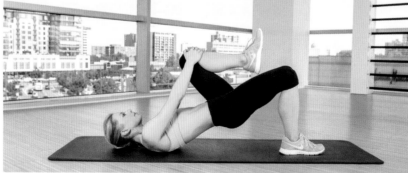

Contrary to popular belief, the burn that we feel in our muscles during exercise is not directly related to caloric burn or the amount of fat that is being burned. Just because you feel a burn in your abdominal muscles during a crunch, it does not mean that your body is burning fat in that area. That sensation in your muscles is actually an indication that your body is out of its quickest form of energy called adenosine triphosphate (ATP), and it needs to slow down or stop doing the exercise in order to produce more. ATP is the building block of energy for all physical activity. In order for your muscles to contract and your body to move, they must have a steady supply of ATP. Because they have a very limited supply on hand at any given time, our bodies use metabolic pathways to produce more ATP on the fly. There are three metabolic pathways: adenosine triphosphate–phosphocreatine (ATP-PC), glycolysis, and aerobic ATP production. Depending on the intensity and duration of your workout, your body might utilize energy from all three pathways. What you need to know for the purposes of fat loss is that the higher you get your heart rate, the more these metabolic pathways will burn calories. It's tempting to base the effectiveness of a workout on how much "burn" you feel in the muscles, but it's the intensity and duration of the workout that will truly determine how many calories—and therefore how much fat—you are melting away.

Where exactly does core work fall on the spectrum of calorie burning? Unfortunately, most traditional core exercises are not scorching a lot of calories. You can do crunches all day long and see no change to the fat you store around your midsection because your heart rate isn't high enough, which means you aren't burning calories at a significant rate. Again, it might *feel* as if you're working hard because your ab muscles are burning and you can't do more than 20 reps, but if you were to wear a heart rate monitor during crunches, it would show that your heart rate rarely gets above 90 beats per minute. When it comes to burning fat and losing weight, your heart rate is the prime indicator of success. It's simple math: The higher your heart rate, the more calories you burn, and the more calories you burn, the more fat you lose. One pound of fat is equal to 3,500 calories, so you need to focus on exercises that will get your heart rate high enough to burn the maximum amount of calories in the shortest amount of time.

The higher your heart rate, the more calories you burn, and the more calories you burn, the more fat you lose.

CALORIES BURNED DURING DIFFERENT WORKOUTS

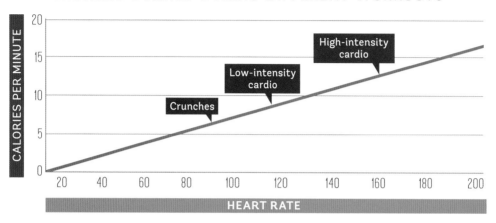

How will you know which types of workouts are maximizing your fat loss? In 2005, the *Journal of Sports Sciences* published a study that outlined an equation to predict the number of calories burned per hour based on your average heart rate.[2] We can apply this equation to different types of sculpting and cardio routines to determine which ones deliver the best results. As the oft-used adage goes: Don't work harder, work smarter.

Let's take the old crunches-based core routine as a starting point for caloric burn. If we assume an average heart rate of 90 beats per minute (which is the heart rate most of my clients exhibit while doing crunches), a 40-year-old female who weighs 160 pounds will burn approximately 195 calories in an hour. You could burn that many calories in 20 minutes by doing a moderate jog. Plus, when was the last time you did crunches for

an hour? Most of us can last about 1 minute, which translates into 3.25 calories burned—that's less than the calorie content of a breath mint. This is one of the myriad reasons why you won't see standard crunches in my Core Envy sculpting routines. Instead, I've focused on exercises that recruit more of the muscles in the core, therefore burning off calories faster by elevating your heart rate. Keep in mind, however, that in order to truly maximize the fat burn around your belly, these sculpting workouts need to be paired with cardio. Sculpting routines alone cannot ensure optimal caloric burn.

THE TRUTH ABOUT SPOT-REDUCING FAT

We all store fat in different areas of our bodies; women with pear-shaped bodies tend to store more in the hips and thighs, while women with apple-shaped bodies store more in the abdomen and upper arms. When you want to reduce fat in a specific area of your body, it would seem reasonable to do exercises that work the muscles in that region. So if you want less fat on your thighs, you do lunges; if you want less fat on your arms, you do biceps curls; and if you want to burn off that spare tire, you do core exercises. Seems perfectly logical, doesn't it? Unfortunately, this approach to fat reduction is simply false. The reason we can't microtarget fat areas is that fat is stored primarily in the form of triglycerides. These triglycerides might tend to collect more in certain areas (such as the abdomen or thighs), but that doesn't mean the muscles of that area are using those specific triglycerides for fuel.

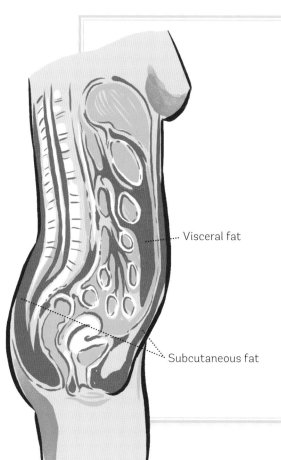

Visceral fat

Subcutaneous fat

IS ALL BELLY FAT
the same?

Fat located beneath the skin—the stuff you can pinch—is called "subcutaneous" fat. This is the same type of fat found on the thighs and upper arms. Fat located near the abdominal organs is called visceral fat, and it is associated with an increased risk of type II diabetes, colorectal cancer, high levels of LDL cholesterol, high blood pressure, and a host of other ailments.[3]

Visceral fat is also the main culprit behind a bulging tummy. The good news is that visceral fat tends to respond quite well to high-intensity interval training and a decrease in consumption of calories, especially sugar and refined carbohydrates.

When we need energy to move, our body will call upon the stored energy in our fat cells and convert that energy into fuel that our muscles can use. Just because we have fat cells in our stomach doesn't mean our body will choose those particular fat cells to convert to energy when we're doing core exercises. In short, the fat cells in our stomach don't "belong" to the muscles of the stomach. The body will pull energy from fat cells in many different areas of the body and will use that fuel to help power whatever activity we are doing. For this reason, the key to burning fat as quickly as possible is to choose activities that burn the highest number of calories, in turn eliminating the highest amount of fat. In the next chapter, we will look at which types of workouts are the most effective for burning fat calories, and we'll examine why manipulating your heart rate is the key to losing belly fat.

START WITH A POSTURE MAKEOVER

A few years ago I worked with a woman who was very concerned about building her abdominal muscles back up after two pregnancies. I immediately noticed how rounded her shoulders were and that her posture was making her stomach stick out enough that you might begin to wonder if she were still pregnant. She looked down at her stomach and exclaimed, "See? Ever since I had kids, I have this horrible pooch that won't go away!" I promptly pulled her shoulders back and told her to lift her chest up 3 inches. Voilà! Her dreaded "mommy tummy" disappeared immediately. She was shocked but came to the realization that she had started slouching thanks to her daily routine of breast-feeding, carrying babies, and being chronically sleep-deprived. I started her on a program that focused on strengthening not only the abdominal muscles but also those of the upper back and midback. Her posture improved dramatically, the mommy tummy went away, and her confidence skyrocketed.

The problem of poor posture is not restricted to mothers and older women. Over the past decade, I've noticed a significant increase in the number of women who come to me with extremely poor posture. As poor posture becomes more and more prevalent, our collective memory of good posture fades away. The ramifications go far beyond vanity and a belly pooch. When the spine is excessively rounded forward for long periods of time, ischemic tissue (tissue that no longer has oxygen flow to it) will develop in the area and contribute to the irreversible curvature of the spine. In addition, poor posture can interfere with the brain's ability to communicate with the muscles (by putting pressure on the spinal column), can cause joint and muscle injuries, and can even lead to painful trigger points from overused muscles.

Are you SLOUCHING?

Take a look at your profile in a mirror and compare your natural posture with the illustrations shown here. The position of your head will have a domino effect on the rest of your spine. You can experience this by pushing your chin forward 6 inches, which should cause your upper back and shoulders to round forward and your chest cavity to collapse.

Notice that if you have poor posture, it is likely that your shoulders are slumped and your hips are tucked under in a way that makes your gluteals look weak and untoned, which in turn makes your stomach look bigger. Now move your body into the opposite position, which is called a back extension. The abdominal muscles immediately become elongated and flatter, the shoulders pull back and create an opening in the chest, and the hips move into a slight anterior pelvic tilt (pushed backward), which helps the gluteals look round and toned.

When your mother harped on you to stand up straight and pull your shoulders back, she should have mentioned that good posture makes your chest, abs, and butt more attractive. Now, I'm not talking about an exaggerated position like that of a gymnast saluting the judges. You want to find the natural posture that helps you look great and allows your spinal column to rest in its optimal position.

There are four primary regions of the spine, and each one exhibits a curve called either "lordosis" or "kyphosis." If the natural curve becomes exaggerated, it can result in postural distortions. Because of the ever increasing use of computers and cell phones and time spent sitting and slouching, the presence and severity of postural distortions are growing at an alarming rate. While this sounds serious, most postural distortions can be corrected by strengthening the muscles of the core—especially those that are chronically underutilized. You will notice that the core routines in this book focus heavily on exercises that use the muscles on the sides and back of the core. This is not an accident. We have already established that most traditional core routines focus on strengthening the already dominant rectus abdominis. In contrast, the routines in this book work on elongating the rectus abdominis while strengthening the deep abdominals and the muscles responsible for spinal rotation and stabilization. Oh, and at the same time, the routines will make your core chiseled. Not a bad combo.

The take-home lesson is that how you train your body to move during workouts will affect how your body moves during real life. If you lie on the ground and repeatedly train your shoulders to crunch down toward your hips, when you stand up, your body will naturally move into this pattern as well. Likewise, if you push your chin and head forward during movements such as crunches, push-ups, or lunges, then you are training your chin and head to push forward while you stand and walk.

Many women believe that the common progression to poor posture is collateral damage of the aging process, an unavoidable consequence of a lifetime trying to combat gravity. Although conditions such as scoliosis are largely hereditary and therefore unpreventable, they are rare (occurring in 2 to 3 percent of the US population). The vast majority of poor-posture culprits are actually quite treatable through regular exercise. In fact, regular exercise helps maintain proper alignment of the spine and also helps slow the loss of bone density. Rest assured that the exercises in this book are designed not only to give you an enviable core but to keep the muscles around your spine healthy and strong, giving you the added benefit of an ideal, sexy posture.

AN ENVIABLE CORE FEELS GOOD

In addition to helping your posture, a strong core can play a critical role in keeping you pain-free, specifically in the low back. If you've experienced low-back pain, you've probably been told that improving your core strength can help alleviate your discomfort. I've had multiple clients come to me claiming that they've been working on their core strength at the behest of a doctor. With no

How is your DYNAMIC POSTURE?

Not only do we need to maintain good static posture while we're standing or sitting but we also need to keep this posture during movement. Dynamic posture, or the position of our bodies during movement, is just as important as static posture, but it's often overlooked.

One of the quickest ways I can tell whether or not a client has good dynamic posture is to have her do a squat with her arms held straight up overhead. If she collapses forward during the squat, rounding her shoulders and letting the chest fall toward the legs, that's a telltale indicator that the core muscles aren't strong enough to support the spinal column. In other words, the dynamic posture of the spine is compromised.

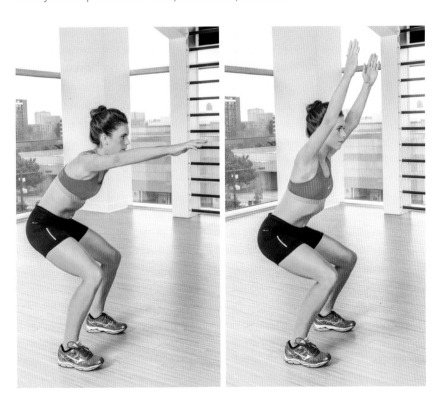

specific instructions beyond "improve core strength," you might leave the doctor's office and immediately begin a program of crunches, twisting crunches, side crunches, and several other movements that involve lying on your back and bringing your torso toward your knees. After weeks or months of following this protocol, chances are high that you're not only still suffering from low-back pain but may actually be experiencing an increase in symptoms. How can this be? What went wrong?

In order to understand why crunches can actually exacerbate low-back pain, we must first look at the basic structure and function of the spine. Our spinal column consists of the spinal cord, the spinal nerves, 33 vertebrae (bones), and 24 intervertebral discs that provide padding between each vertebra. The intervertebral discs live only between the vertebrae of the cervical, thoracic, and lumbar spinal regions; we have 9 additional fused vertebrae in the sacrum and coccyx that aren't separated by discs.

The integrity of the intervertebral discs is crucial to maintaining a healthy, pain-free spine. If the position of the discs is compromised in any way, then you are in danger of experiencing a bulging, herniated, or slipped disc. Almost 90 percent of disc injuries occur in the lumbar (low-back) area of the spine, most frequently between L4 and L5 and L5 and S1.[4] As you can see from the figure (page 23), when a disc herniation occurs, the gel-like substance in the middle of the disc (nucleus pulposus) pushes its way outside the disc and starts to press against nerve roots. Pressure on a nerve root can cause debilitating pain that can run all the way down the back or side of the leg.

The two main causes of disc herniation are normal wear and tear (also called degenerative disc disease) and a traumatic event. Normal wear and tear on the spine happens every day, as we call upon the discs to cushion the spine while we bend, twist, rotate, and carry heavy objects. Over time, the discs will start to wear down and lose their ability to effectively withstand these forces. We can help maintain and improve upon the health of our spinal discs by enhancing good posture and good muscle tone; this is where core strength comes into play.

The key to building the type of core necessary to prevent low-back pain is to choose exercises that help maintain the spine in its neutral position. In its proper position, the lumbar spine should exhibit a slight lordotic curve of 4 to 7 degrees in men and 7 to 10 degrees in women. In other words, your low back should have a very subtle arch or extension. When the lumber spine is tucked under, it goes into flexion, which forces the spine into an unnatural position and puts undue stress on those crucial intervertebral discs. Abdominal crunches not only compromise the position of your spine but also force the cervical (neck) spine into an excessively flexed position, causing

ALL ABOUT THE SPINE

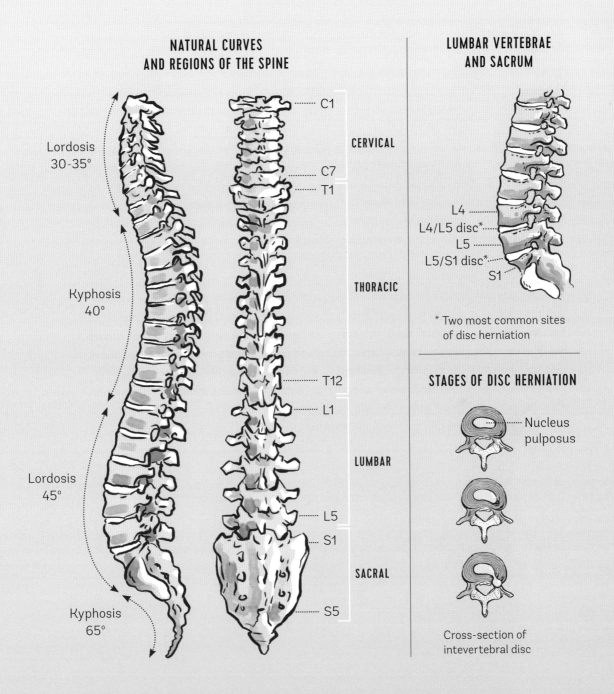

NATURAL CURVES AND REGIONS OF THE SPINE

Lordosis 30-35°

Kyphosis 40°

Lordosis 45°

Kyphosis 65°

C1

CERVICAL

C7
T1

THORACIC

T12

L1

LUMBAR

L5
S1

SACRAL

S5

LUMBAR VERTEBRAE AND SACRUM

L4
L4/L5 disc*
L5
L5/S1 disc*
S1

* Two most common sites of disc herniation

STAGES OF DISC HERNIATION

Nucleus pulposus

Cross-section of intevertebral disc

neck and upper-back pain. Needless to say, avoiding improper spinal positions should be a priority in any exercise routine.

WHY YOU SHOULD DO CORE WORK

With all these facts and statistics showing that most core exercises (particularly the traditional crunch-based routines) are not, in fact, going to create the enviable core we desire, why should we do core exercises at all? If doing high-intensity cardio burns fat more effectively than crunches, why wouldn't you just do cardio all day long and ditch the brutal core routines? Here's why: Working the core in a functional, progressive manner will give you nice, lean muscles that will be on display once that layer of fat is burned off by doing cardio and cleaning up your diet. You don't want to spend months burning off that spare tire to reveal, well, nothing underneath.

While core exercises are not the most effective way to burn subcutaneous and visceral fat off your belly, they *are* the answer to toning the muscles underneath. As stated earlier, spot-reducing fat from your body is not realistic, but spot-toning your muscles most certainly is. For example, you can absolutely make the muscles in your legs stronger and more toned by doing lunges and squats; this maxim holds true for any muscle in the body. Putting repetitive stress on a muscle causes positive adaptations in those muscle fibers that range from improved cardiovascular efficiency to increased bone density and neuromuscular control. The bottom line is that if you put repetitive stress on your core muscles by doing the sculpting exercises in this book, you will improve the strength, power, endurance, and coordination of those muscles. All of these benefits are just lovely side effects of sculpting a gorgeous, enviable core!

I stopped doing crunches and finally got the kick-ass core I always wanted!

I STARTED THE CORE ENVY PLAN while I was flying all over the country for interviews to get into a medical residency program. I figured if the plan fit my hectic schedule, I could realistically stick with it long-term. My midsection has always been my Achilles heel, so to speak, and I had been including lots of crunches in my workout routine. If I only had 20 minutes to work out, I would choose crunches over cardio because I honestly believed it would give me better results. The thought of skipping crunches when my tummy was my trouble area seemed ridiculous to me . . . until I was introduced to the Core Envy program. The explanation of what types of core work are effective made sense to me as a doctor, so I decided to give it a shot.

The plan was super-easy to follow because it doesn't require any equipment or a gym membership—I was able to complete all the core sculpting routines and the cardio work-outs at home or in my hotel room. Sometimes I went outside to do the cardio, but there were several days when I just banged out 18 minutes of jumping jacks or dancing in order to get my heart rate up to the prescribed level.

Initially, I worried about whether the diet would work for me because I don't have control over what's put in front of me at most of my meals—sometimes it's pizza and breadsticks for lunch, and I have to decide whether to eat it or go hungry . . . or at least that's what I've always told myself. If you have no choice in what's put in front of you, then it's not your fault if you can't make good decisions, right? That was my excuse, and I'd been using it for a long time. Allison's plan taught me that I always have some degree of control over what I eat; I just have to be prepared. In other words, I began assuming that the food put in front of me was going to be unhealthy, so I prepared by packing snacks in my purse like healthy bars, pieces of fruit, nuts, and hard-boiled eggs. These items became as essential to my leaving-the-house routine as grabbing my wallet and keys.

By the end of 8 weeks, I had lost 2 inches off my stomach, and my stubborn muffin top was gone. More importantly, I finally understand how to structure my workout routine and my diet to get the results I want in my midsection. They say that knowledge is power, and I'm feeling very powerful thanks to the Core Envy program!

Step 2: CARDIO WORKOUTS that MELT FAT

WE HAVE EXPLORED THE SCIENCE behind sculpting gorgeous core muscles and what types of movements and workouts are the most effective for accomplishing this goal, but those muscles will never be seen if you don't burn off the layer of fat that's sitting on top. What's the most effective method for burning up that spare tire? Cardio workouts. That's right—going for a run will actually do more to burn off abdominal fat than banging out 500 crunches. While the core exercises found in this book will likely get your heart rate higher than the core work you've been doing, the calories burned during a sculpting routine are not enough; the cardio workouts I've put together for you will pick up the slack in the calorie-burning department and ensure that your hard-earned core muscles aren't hiding under a stubborn layer of fat. By incorporating a mix of cardio workouts into your program, you'll achieve the perfect combination of fat burning and muscle sculpting!

BREAK OUT OF THE FAT-BURNING ZONE

One of the most deep-seated and fiercely argued tenets of cardio work is that in order to burn fat, you should always be working in the "fat-burning zone." If you've ever been on a cardio machine at a health club, you've seen those nifty little guides that relay the supposed effects of different heart rate zones. With words such as "Maximum Fat Burn Zone" plastered all over lower heart rates, it's no wonder that we've all been seduced into thinking that the only way to burn that stubborn fat off is to keep our heart rates low and steady. This is why many of us insist on setting the treadmill at a brisk walking pace and staying on it for as long as possible. Heaven forbid we get our heart rates too high and enter the "Danger Zone"!

The concept of the "fat-burning zone" is based on the premise that your body burns a greater percentage of calories from fat when it's working at lower heart rates. If we consider this concept alone, you might choose the low-intensity workout. To complete a 30-minute workout at a low intensity, a 130-pound woman can get 50 percent of the energy she needs from fat. If she were instead to do a high-intensity workout for 30 minutes, just 40 percent of the calories burned would come from fat.

But take a closer look and you will see that the high-intensity workout actually burns more total fat calories—12 percent more. The bottom line? For the same amount of time (in this case 30 minutes), you burn more total calories, and you burn more total fat calories during a high-intensity workout than during a low-intensity workout. Don't get caught up in the percentage of total calories that come from fat. You need to burn more calories, and more calories from fat, and the scientifically proven way to accomplish this is through high-intensity interval workouts, not "low and slow" workouts.

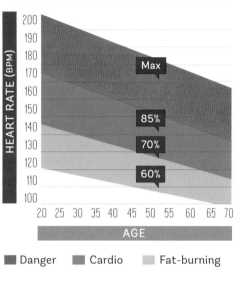

TRADITIONAL TRAINING GUIDE

■ Danger   ■ Cardio   ■ Fat-burning

Still not convinced? Maybe this fact will get your attention: Consistently working out at a low intensity can actually train your body to store fat. You read that correctly. If you consistently perform low-intensity exercise (that is, at a low heart rate), your body will adapt by beginning to store fat so that it can complete the next bout of exercise more effectively. This scenario is called "metabolic efficiency," and it's the ultimate catch-22 of exercising.[1] Being more efficient at anything seems desirable, but an efficient metabolism will get in the way of your goals.

While efficiency is a desirable endpoint for many pursuits in life, it is not the most effective way for your body to burn fat in a sustainable method. Consider what happens to the body when you practice for a specific

If you consistently do low-intensity cardio workouts, *your body will adapt and begin to store fat* so that it can complete the next bout of exercise more effectively. This is called *metabolic efficiency.*

type of activity or sport: You spend countless hours repeating the same movements or the same types of motions so that your body becomes better at them, and eventually you can perform at the same level but with less effort. Because the human body is such an adaptable machine, it will find the easiest way to accomplish a task and follow that route. It's essentially the body's way of always choosing the path of least resistance. This is good news for performance (you'll get better at whatever activity you practice), but it's bad news for your metabolism.

I experienced this phenomenon when I was a sophomore in college and was trying to shed the 15 pounds I had gained freshman year. I did my research and decided that distance running was the solution: It burns lots of calories, requires no equipment besides a pair of shoes, and can be performed anywhere. Perfect, I thought—this was my new weight-loss method! I grew up playing team sports, which led me to assume that picking up a new sport would be a breeze—never mind that I had absolutely zero experience with endurance sports. My longest run at that point in my life had been from one end of the basketball court to the other. Realizing that I might need to slowly work at building my endurance, I decided to run for just 20 minutes my first time out.

CALORIC BREAKDOWN FOR LOW- VS. HIGH-INTENSITY EXERCISE

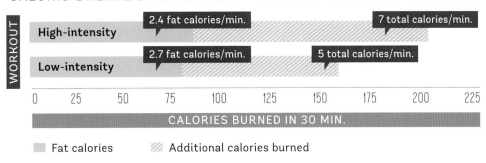

Precisely 3 minutes into that first run, I found myself doubled over with a side cramp and gasping for air. This new form of exercise was taxing my body in unfamiliar ways! Though it was challenging—often to the point of complete emotional and mental failure—I stuck with it, and six months later, I ran my first half-marathon. I also cleaned up my diet, so by the time that half-marathon arrived, I had lost not only the 15 pounds I had gained my freshman year but also another 10 that fell off without any extra effort. Having found a formula that worked for me, I hit repeat and became extremely loyal to the endurance run. Those long, slow runs were the staple of my workout regimen for years, and my strategy continued to work . . . until it didn't.

After a few years, my body began to adapt to this regimen, and the runs no longer had the same effect. I became efficient at running, and despite the fact that I was running longer distances, the pounds started to creep back on. Frustrated, I made the mistake that we have all made in many areas of life: If something isn't working, then do more of the same thing, and you'll get better results! I increased my mileage, eventually getting to a point where I was running almost 40 miles a week. But as my miles increased, so did the number on the scale.

Convinced that the additional pounds were from increased muscle mass, I had my body fat tested through a dual-energy X-ray

HOW DISTANCE RUNNING CAN CAUSE WEIGHT GAIN

- ▶ Once your metabolism masters steady-state runs, it burns fewer calories for each workout.

- ▶ If your training doesn't include high-intensity work, you are missing an opportunity to boost your metabolism for the 24-hour period following your workout. Long, slow runs burn very few calories after the workout is over.

- ▶ Runners are notorious for overtraining, and the subsequent spike in cortisol triggers the body to store fat in your abdominal area.

absorptiometry (DEXA) scan, which reveals in great detail the areas of your body that are housing fat and muscle. The DEXA scan has a very small margin of error, so I knew the numbers would be reliable. The results were sobering: I had gained body fat, and it was concentrated primarily on my hips and upper legs, the very areas that I was working relentlessly through my long runs. That was the day I realized I had to make significant changes to my exercise and diet regimen. By stubbornly following a program that had worked in the past, I was now sabotaging my fitness and my waistline. I did some

POST-EXERCISE BENEFITS OF HIGH-INTENSITY TRAINING

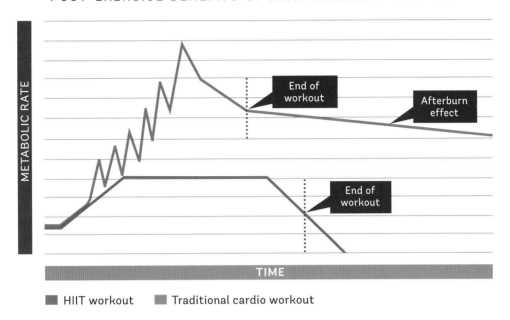

METABOLIC RATE

End of workout

Afterburn effect

End of workout

TIME

■ HIIT workout   ■ Traditional cardio workout

research, I talked to my colleagues, and I came up with a game plan: Ditch the long, low-intensity cardio and start focusing on high-intensity intervals and strength training. My new goal was to throw my body into a state of metabolic confusion.

THE ADVANTAGE OF METABOLIC CONFUSION

Metabolic confusion is the opposite of metabolic efficiency. By regularly switching up the duration, intensity, and type of exercise you're doing, you can keep your metabolism on its toes. When your body doesn't know what type of workout is coming next, it doesn't have the opportunity to

burn fewer calories in order to complete the task at hand. Instead, your body is forced to react to the ever-changing stimuli of new workouts and therefore will burn a higher amount of calories. Studies show that high-intensity interval training (HIIT) is the most effective form of exercise to achieve metabolic confusion and burn abdominal visceral fat.[2]

What constitutes a HIIT workout? Any activity that spikes your heart rate up to about 70 percent of its maximum for a short period of time, then allows you to recover at a lower heart rate, then spikes your heart rate up again. If you were to graph your heart rate, it might look a rising series of peaks and valleys.

The beauty of HIIT workouts is that they require less time. One of the most-cited reasons for missing a workout is lack of time; I've heard this excuse on countless occasions over the years from my clients. You can bang out a fat-burning workout in a surprisingly short amount of time. In fact, the workouts that I've created for the Core Envy program (pages 167–185) range from 16 to 36 minutes. I'm guessing that you have 36 minutes in your day that you could devote to getting leaner, tighter, and healthier. According to the US Bureau of Labor, Americans over the age of 15 spend an average of 2.8 hours a day watching television, which is more than five times longer than the time required for a HIIT workout.[3] Don't want to give up your favorite episodes to sweat it out? Watch TV while you exercise! HIIT sessions don't require you to do any specific type of movement; they require only that you get your heart rate up to a certain level. You could accomplish this by running, cycling, dancing, hitting a boxing bag, jumping rope, or any number of other movements that can be performed in the comfort of your home while simultaneously watching your favorite shows.

The effectiveness of HIIT workouts is because of a phenomenon known as excess postexercise oxygen consumption (EPOC). After a workout, your body will continue to consume oxygen for a certain amount of time in order to bring your body back into its resting state. The more oxygen your body consumes, and the longer it does this, the more calories you will burn. As you know, more calories burned equals more pounds lost, which equals a tighter tummy for you. The key letter in the acronym is "P" for postexercise. This means that not only are you burning fat during your workout but you will also continue to burn calories and fat long after your workout has ended.

A substantial number of studies have been done around EPOC; many compare the exact amount of calories burned postexercise during different types of workouts.[4] Workouts that involve bouts of high intensity clearly provide a much higher caloric burn both during the workout and for up to 48 hours afterward. More specifically, workouts that require your heart rate to get to 70 percent of its maximum seem to be the most effective. For this reason, every HIIT workout I've created for the Core Envy program targets that magical 70 percent threshold.

WHY HIIT WORKOUTS ARE BEST FOR TARGETING ABDOMINAL FAT

- ▶ You will burn more total calories and more fat calories.

- ▶ Your metabolism will remain elevated for up to 48 hours postworkout.

If you're concerned that performing high-intensity exercise is too aggressive for your current state of fitness, remember that heart rate is relative. My 70 percent threshold will look much different than yours, which will look different than that of a professional athlete, and so on. If walking up a flight of stairs elevates your heart rate and makes it difficult for you to talk, then that is likely your 70 percent. As you complete the Core Envy program and your cardio conditioning increases, your body will adapt, and soon you'll be able to walk up those stairs faster, perhaps even progressing toward a gentle jog. By the end of the 8-week program, your 70 percent will look and feel much different than it did when you started. How can you tell when you've reached 70 percent of your maximum heart rate? Don't worry; I will explain how to find your target heart rates in the "Core Envy Cardio Workouts" chapter. You'll become a master at manipulating your own heart rate after just a few workouts, which will ensure that you're burning the maximum amount of calories in the shortest amount of time.

HOW STRESS IMPACTS YOUR WAISTLINE

If you have long suspected that stress is contributing to the pounds around your midsection, you're right. As if we weren't already fighting an uphill battle to stay fit (demanding jobs, family obligations,

unhealthy food lurking at every turn), now we have to add stress to the mix! Americans are under more stress than ever. According to the 2013 report "Stress in America" conducted by the American Psychological Association, 52 percent of adults say that their stress levels have increased over the past five years, and the average stress level is 5.3 (on a scale of 1 to 10), higher than what is considered healthy or manageable. One ironic point about our ever-increasing stress levels is that 57 percent of adults report that exercising lowers their stress levels and makes them feel better, yet only 17 percent of Americans actually do some form of exercise on a daily basis.[5] Furthermore, stress is cited as a reason for why Americans are skipping workouts, which in turn creates more stress, and thus the cycle continues.

So how can stress actually contribute to the girth of your waistline? It's due to the release of a hormone called cortisol. If you experience normal day-to-day stress, your body is equipped to fight it off by releasing the hormones epinephrine or norepinephrine—better known as the "fight or flight" hormones. But when you experience chronic, relentless stress, your body begins to release a hormone called cortisol. When too much cortisol is present in the body, it triggers what is known as the cortisol cascade.

The cortisol cascade essentially prompts the body to store fat in order to protect your organs, and since the major organs of the body are located in the trunk (except your skin, which is actually the largest organ of the body), that is where the majority of the fat deposits will congregate. These fat cells will search out and surround your organs, resulting in increased visceral fat. Another term for visceral fat is "belly fat," which describes the area of the body in which this type of fat resides. Visceral fat is much more dangerous than subcutaneous fat (the type that sit right below the skin, typically found on your thighs and arms) because it has the ability to travel deep within the body and surround the organs, creating a marbling effect. This type of fat places you at a much greater risk for developing some serious diseases and conditions that you don't want to deal with, such as type II diabetes, coronary artery disease, metabolic syndrome, and sleep apnea. While visceral fat typically makes your belly larger, it can accumulate regardless of whether or not you are overweight. In fact, you can have a high level of visceral fat and still be at a normal weight according to medical charts.

STRATEGIES FOR REDUCING VISCERAL FAT

We know that excess levels of the hormone cortisol can trigger a cascade effect that will cause the body to store fat in the abdominal region, but what can we do to get rid of it? There are several tried-and-true methods of lowering your cortisol levels, one of which is to engage in regular high-intensity bouts of exercise. Because visceral fat is located deep within the abdomen, it can often be more stubborn than your run-of-the-mill subcutaneous body fat. Many clients have come to me with the goal of losing a persistent paunch, and the single most effective workout strategy is HIIT. These types of workouts produce the biggest results in the shortest amount of time; combined with my Core Envy nutrition plan, you can expect to see results in just a few weeks. By the end of 8 weeks, not only will you be well on your way to a tighter tummy, but your fitness levels will improve as well, allowing you to push your workouts to the next level.

CORTISOL CASCADE

Cortisol releases fatty acids into the bloodstream.

These fatty acids relocate to the deep abdomen in order to protect the organs. This causes "visceral obesity."

Fat deposition is enhanced in order to protect the body.

Do you have unhealthy
AMOUNTS OF VISCERAL FAT?

A DEXA scan, MRI, or InBody scan of your abdomen are the best ways to quantify visceral fat, but since most of us don't have the time or resources to make one of those scans happen, a much easier method is simply to measure the circumference of your belly. Use a tailor's tape or another flexible form of measurement. Place it at the top of your hip bone and complete a circle around your waist, being sure to keep the tape level. For women, a waist circumference indicating an unhealthy amount of visceral fat is over 35 inches (as compared to 40 inches for men).

If your waist measurement is over the prescribed limit, you are twice as likely to face the risks associated with visceral abdominal fat.[6] In other words, a high level of fat in your abdomen is not only unsightly but also deadly.

At the back of the book you'll find a chart for tracking your body measurements (see page 188). Don't be discouraged if your numbers are off the mark. Be diligent in following the program and tracking your measurements, and you will begin to see the progress.

The only caveat about HIIT is that more is not always better. The reason high-intensity exercise is effective is because it taxes the body, which causes a release of good hormones that will help fight abdominal fat, but only to a point. When the body is asked to perform a challenging task such as exercise, it actually creates stress and causes your body to release growth hormones and testosterone.[7] These hormones actively reduce adipose tissue (fat) and help to reduce the storage of abdominal fat, making your body leaner and less likely to hold on to additional fat. There is a limit, however, to how much stress the body can handle; if you tax your body too often and too intensely, you will pass the threshold of good stress and cross over into the bad stress zone, causing a release of that dreaded cortisol. In order to avoid this scenario, it's important to give your body time to recover between HIIT workouts, ideally 48 hours. For this reason,

EFFECTS *of* OVERTRAINING

The Core Envy program is designed sensibly to avoid overtraining. However, if you think you are at risk of pushing too hard, be alert for the following signs.

PSYCHOLOGICAL	PHYSICAL
Anger	Increased chance of injury
Fatigue	Muscle soreness
Sleep problems	Increased cortisol levels (fat enhancer)
Depression	Decreased testosterone levels (fat reducer)

I have created weekly workout schedules (page 167) that allow ample time for your body to recover after a HIIT workout but keep you working out consistently. On the days when you aren't doing a HIIT workout, you'll be focusing on lower-intensity cardio and sculpting exercises for your core. This approach allows you to reap the benefits of doing cardio on a regular basis without causing too much stress.

One of the best side effects of a HIIT workout is the endorphin high that often kicks in as you push through those intense intervals. A rush of endorphins through the body will give you not only the physical stamina to complete the workout but also the emotional motivation to continue chasing that high. It might be the closest you will ever come to actually feeling like you can fly!

I stopped doing hours of cardio and finally toned up my abs.

A FEW YEARS AGO I decided to reach out to a trainer because I was doing hours and hours of cardio and my body wasn't changing. A friend recommended Allison, and when I scheduled my first appointment, she requested that I show up with a journal of my food and exercise from the past week. She went through it and told me I needed to cut back on my endurance cardio (I was averaging 2 hours a day of something low and slow for heart rate), increase my sculpting routines, and reduce the number of calories I was consuming. This seemed totally illogical to me! How was I going to lose the stubborn fat sitting on my tummy if I wasn't working out during every spare minute of my day?!

I decided to commit to her approach for two months because I really did want to see change in my body, and my long hikes and endless walks just weren't cutting it. I stopped waking up at 4 a.m. to work out (that was nice!) and instead increased my sleep, which actually helped me feel less hungry and more focused. I did the HIIT workouts a few times a week, incorporated the sculpting routines she gave me, and made a major commitment to rid my diet of sugar. Two weeks into this new program I was already feeling lighter; by four weeks my pants were noticeably looser; and by the end of the 8 weeks I had lost 7 pounds of fat, 3 inches off my waist, and another 2 inches off my hips. I'm hooked on the Core Envy program—it's allowed me to get the results I want by working out less, which I thought was impossible!

Step 3: EATING for
WEIGHT LOSS

THERE ARE TWO BASIC GUIDELINES for the Core Envy Diet: (1) Eat fewer calories, and (2) make those calories highly nutritious. If you can do this on a regular basis, you will not only lose inches around your waistline, you'll also reap the health benefits of being well nourished. I don't just want you to have an enviable core; I want you to have an enviable core that is part of a vibrant, energetic, and healthy body. You may have started this program solely to look better, but if you implement the Core Envy Diet, you will also establish lasting and meaningful habits around food that will help reduce your risk of chronic illness and disease.

RULE 1: EAT FEWER CALORIES

The basic science of weight loss demands that the calories you consume (also known as energy) be less than the calories you burn. This is called a caloric deficit. In order to make sure you're creating a daily caloric deficit, you need to understand exactly how to calculate the calories in versus calories out. Estimates simply won't suffice, and here's why: If you consume 100 calories a day more than you burn, you will end up gaining 10 pounds over the course of a year. You read that correctly—eating 100 extra calories a day for a year can drastically impact your waistline. If you think you're already aware of how many calories you consume, you might want to check your math. According to the most recent data released by the US Department of Agriculture (USDA), Americans consume an average of 2,569 calories per day, and the majority of these calories come from carbohydrate, sugar, and fat (see figure).[3] Unfortunately, this consumption far exceeds the calories needed to meet the energy demands of a typical American. Let's look at an example: Elizabeth is 40 years old, is 5 feet 5 inches tall, weighs 150 pounds, and typically exercises three days a week at a moderate intensity. Given her age, sex, weight, and activity level, Elizabeth should be consuming 1,851 calories a day in order to maintain her current weight (I'll walk you through this calculation in the next few pages). Every calorie over that 1,851 mark will result in weight gain over time.

Calculating Daily Calories for Weight Loss

We know that most Americans are eating too many calories and not moving enough to burn them off. But how do you find out the number of calories you personally need to consume for weight loss? You start by determining how many calories your body will burn on its own just to maintain its essential body functions. This baseline calorie expenditure is known as the resting metabolic rate (RMR, sometimes referred to as resting energy expenditure, or REE), and it is the number of calories the body would burn if it were at rest for 24 hours. In other words, your RMR is the amount of calories you need to consume on a daily basis in order to maintain

TYPICAL DAILY CALORIC CONSUMPTION

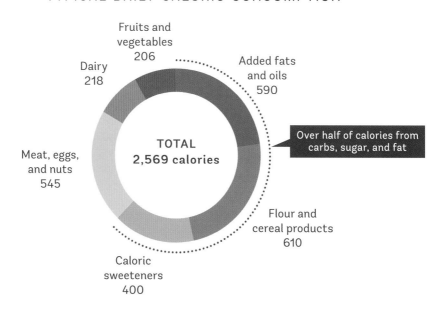

Fruits and vegetables
206

Added fats and oils
590

Dairy
218

TOTAL
2,569 calories

Over half of calories from carbs, sugar, and fat

Meat, eggs, and nuts
545

Flour and cereal products
610

Caloric sweeteners
400

your weight if you are currently leading a sedentary lifestyle. There are countless equations that calculate your RMR, but in the fitness industry the Mifflin equation remains the gold standard.[4]

Once you have completed the Mifflin equation, take the resulting number and multiply it by your level of activity in order to determine the true number of calories you burn on a daily basis. For the purposes of this program, your activity factor should reflect the specific cardio exercise program you plan to follow. For example, if you are not feeling very fit entering into the program, you might want to predominantly focus on the Level 1 cardio routines, so you would use an activity factor of 1.375. If you have a decent fitness base and want to take on a bigger challenge, the Level 2 or Level 3 program will be a better fit, so use the corresponding activity factor.

Why can't we just take
A PILL TO LOSE WEIGHT?

According to a recent survey, one in three American dieters has used supplements to help aid weight loss. The same study showed that most people had no idea that these supplements are unregulated by the US Food and Drug Administration (FDA) and that some have serious side effects, including depression, nausea, and cardiac events.[1]

The FDA has a long history of approving and then recalling prescription weight-loss medications. In 1947, methamphetamine was the first drug approved but was later severely restricted due to concerns about side effects. Over the decades, scores of pills have been temporarily approved, then later recalled once evidence of cardiac failure emerged. Of the weight-loss drugs that are now currently on the FDA's list, studies clearly show that they are effective only when combined with diet and exercise. Furthermore, once usage of any pill is stopped, most of the weight returns within one year.[2]

The bottom line is that eating less and moving more is still the safest, most effective method for losing weight and keeping it off.

HOW TO FIND YOUR RESTING METABOLIC RATE

$$\big[10 \times \text{weight in kg}\big]$$

then add

$$\big[6.25 \times \text{height in cm}\big]$$

then subtract

$$\big[5 \times \text{age}\big]$$

then subtract **161**

To calculate kg, multiply your weight in pounds by 0.45.

To calculate cm, multiply your height in inches by 2.54.

The Mifflin equation is the gold standard for finding your RMR. Visit coreenvybook.com to use our RMR calculator.

For Elizabeth, who is 40 years old, 5 feet 5 inches tall, and 150 pounds, the equation works out like this:

$$\text{RMR} = \big[10 \times 67.5\big] + \big[6.25 \times 165.1\big] - \big[5 \times 40\big] - 161$$

Her resting metabolic rate is 1,346 calories.

HOW TO FIND YOUR WEEKLY ACTIVITY FACTOR

CORE ENVY PROGRAM	ACTIVITY FACTOR
LEVEL 1	1.375
LEVEL 2	1.55
LEVEL 3	1.725

Elizabeth plans to use the Level 1 Core Envy program.
Her RMR is multiplied by the Level 1 activity factor.

$$1{,}346 \times 1.375 = 1{,}851$$

This is her daily caloric goal to maintain her current weight. To lose weight, she will need a daily deficit of 500 calories, which makes her total 1,351 calories. Her target will be 1,400 calories—the daily minimum.

$$\text{RMR} \times \text{Activity Factor} - 500 \text{ Calories} =$$

DAILY CALORIC GOAL FOR WEIGHT LOSS

If your routine will include additional bouts of exercise beyond the workouts in this book, you can err toward a higher activity factor. However, it's always safest to start with a lower activity factor and then add calories back in if necessary. Most of us drastically underestimate how many calories we are consuming, and we also tend to overestimate the number of calories we are burning.

Once you've multiplied your RMR by your activity factor, you will know exactly how many calories you would need to consume each day in order to maintain your current weight. To shed a few pounds (maybe more than a few) and firm up that midsection, you must make sure your actual caloric consumption is lower than this number.

One pound of fat is equal to 3,500 calories, so for every pound of fat you want to lose, you need to create a caloric deficit of 3,500. Based on what we know about calories in versus calories out, this deficit can't be achieved in a day, or even a few days. Assuming you don't dip below the minimum daily intake of 1,400 calories, you need to burn off that additional 3,500 through exercise. To put it into perspective, this would require a daily workout equivalent to running 35 miles. A much more sustainable and realistic approach is to create a daily caloric deficit of 500 calories through a combination of consuming less and moving more. Over the course of a week, this would add up to 1 pound of weight loss. If you have more than 30

DANGERS OF FAD DIETS

▸ Rapid weight loss typically means loss of muscle and water, not fat.

▸ Increased risk of heart disease, cancer, osteoporosis, and liver disease.

▸ Malnutrition due to restriction of major food groups.

pounds to lose, you might find that you initially lose weight much faster than the 1 pound per week pace, but as you approach those last 5–10 pounds, the rate of loss will inevitably slow down. Here's the bottom line: *You can expect to lose 8–16 pounds over the 8 weeks of the Core Envy program, and if you do it right, you will also gain muscle tone and feel great.*

Losing 1 pound a week might sound painstakingly slow—you've probably followed diet plans before that promised much bigger results in a shorter amount of time. In fact, you may have enjoyed rapid weight loss on these types of plans, but I'm guessing that the weight came back, or you wouldn't be reading this book. The truth is, there's no fast, easy method to lose weight and keep it off. Sure, the scale might say that you've lost 5 pounds in 5 days when you follow a highly restrictive diet, but in fact most of that loss won't be fat; it will be water pounds lost through dehydration. If you eat a bagel on day 6, you will magically gain back those 5 pounds you just thought you lost. How is this possible? For every gram of carbohydrate you consume, the body stores 3 to 4 grams of water. That means for every 400 grams of carbohydrate you consume, your body will store 16 ounces (1 pound) of water. By simply cutting out 400 grams of carbs a day, you can "lose" 1 pound on the scale. But again, this is just a reduction in hydration, and hydration is a key factor in long-term weight loss. And long-term weight loss is all about losing fat, not dehydrating your body.

The Lean Muscle Factor

Isn't lean body mass a deciding factor in how many calories your body burns? Countless blogs, fitness articles, and other media claim that muscle burns 50 times more calories than fat. By this estimate, gaining 10 pounds of muscle would increase your resting metabolic rate by 500 calories a day. This is the kind of pseudoscientific dialogue heard in gyms around the world that I like to call "bro science." Although it likely sounds correct, there is equal likelihood that it is complete BS. In this case, the possibility of your metabolic rate being 500 calories higher is alluring, but it's simply not true.

Scientific studies consistently show that 1 pound of muscle burns approximately 6 calories a day at rest, whereas 1 pound of fat burns 2 calories a day at rest.[5] In other words, that 10 pounds of muscle burns only 40 calories a day more than 10 pounds of fat. If you eat two egg whites, one large bite of a bagel, or two tortilla chips, you've

BENEFITS OF LEAN MUSCLE MASS

▸ Muscle looks firmer than fat and takes up less space because it is more dense.

▸ Fat is associated with dramatically high risks of heart disease, type II diabetes, stroke, and dementia. Muscle is not associated with any of these conditions.

▸ Muscle allows you to work harder during your workouts, which in turn produces greater caloric burn, which melts off fat.

already hit the additional energy quota. Not as much as you had thought, is it?

While body composition does have a modest impact on your RMR, it is very difficult to get a true reading of your lean body mass. The most accurate equipment is cost-prohibitive, and more accessible tools are highly variable. The caloric goal you arrived at using the Mifflin equation is the best place to start, and from there you can make small adjustments based on how your body is responding.

The Dangers of Overrestricting Calories

You might find it tempting to commit to a bigger calorie deficit in an effort to lose weight faster on the Core Envy program. If you are like most Americans (30 to 40 pounds overweight and inactive) and

The dangers of consuming less than 1,400 calories a day on a regular basis *far outweigh the initial weight loss.*

you calculate your RMR multiplied by the activity factor, there is a good chance that you came up with 1,600 to 1,700 calories. Knowing that this is the number necessary to maintain her current weight, the ambitious dieter might be tempted to start drastically slashing calories in order to achieve a large deficit for the day. After all, you want to lose weight, and to lose weight you must consume *less* than the calories you need to maintain your current weight. While this idea is technically correct from a mathematical standpoint, the dangers of consuming less than 1,400 calories a day on a regular basis far outweigh the initial weight loss. Studies consistently show that severe calorie restriction actually lowers RMR, sometimes as much as 16 percent.[6] If your RMR is low, that means your body burns fewer calories at rest, and typically your RMR will stay low even if you switch back to eating a healthy number of calories. Worse yet, if you severely restrict calories and experience rapid weight loss, you actually increase your chances that you will gain that weight back.

How to adjust
CALORIC INTAKE for BREAST-FEEDING

If you are currently breast-feeding and are following this plan to drop the baby weight, you will want to add 200–500 calories a day to your RMR. Once you get the go-ahead from your doctor to work out, you can begin the exercise plan—even the high-intensity interval workouts are safe. Just be sure to stay hydrated by drinking at least half your body weight in ounces each day (for a 150-pound woman, that's 75 ounces of water). If you developed a condition known as diastasis recti during your pregnancy, you should explain to your doctor that you would like to follow a program that focuses on working the core muscles and get clearance to perform the core sculpting exercises in this book.

Learning How to Count Calories

As an educated fitness professional, nothing infuriates me more than diet and weight-loss plans that insist that counting calories is not necessary. "No more counting calories, no more measuring your food, just follow this super-restrictive plan and the pounds will fall off!" Assuming you do follow these plans to the letter, you probably will indeed lose weight because the plan has actually counted calories for you! There is absolutely no way to get around the scientific equation of calories in versus calories out. Our bodies burn calories because calories are energy, and we expend this energy every time we move. When you consume more energy than you burn, the body will store that extra energy as fat so that it can convert it back into energy at a later date. The problem is that most of us never get around to burning those stored calories. Instead, we just keep consuming more and more energy (calories) while simultaneously using less and less of it in our daily activity. There is a proven formula for losing weight: Consume fewer calories while simultaneously burning more of them, and you will like the result. So do the math. Keeping track of the calories you eat can be time-consuming and tedious. However, it's the magic bullet that will finally allow you to take control of your body.

SIGNS THAT YOUR CALORIE CONSUMPTION IS TOO LOW

- ▶ Chronic fatigue
- ▶ Mood swings
- ▶ Amenorrhea (cessation of menstrual period)
- ▶ Rapid and sustained weight loss (more than 5 pounds a week for more than 4 weeks)
- ▶ Poor circulation/coldness in fingers and toes
- ▶ Insomnia and other sleep disturbances

The first few weeks of counting calories are always the most labor-intensive, which is why the Core Envy Diet includes sample menus, 100-calorie portions, and a daily log to make keeping track of your calories a breeze. The activity factor used to calculate your daily caloric goal takes into account the energy (or calories) needed for the sculpting and cardio workouts. While I've listed the caloric burn for the cardio workouts in the book, you don't have to worry about totaling "calories out." Simply do the workouts and eat the right foods to hit your daily caloric goal, and you will be on your way to losing weight.

Calories in < calories out = *weight-loss success!*

RULE 2: MAKE CALORIES NUTRITIOUS

Now that you've calculated the number of calories you need to consume each day to lose weight, it's time to focus on the quality of those calories. The Core Envy Diet focuses on a selection of fat-burning foods, with an emphasis on organic fruits and vegetables, lean meats, unsaturated fats, and whole-grain carbohydrates. The plan is straightforward and easy to follow. If you make these foods staples in your diet you will achieve an enviable core. My goal is to get your body and your taste buds used to eating simple, nutritious foods that will not only whittle away your waistline but also nourish your entire system. The foods I selected for the Core Envy program help burn fat because they meet three key requirements:

▸ Highly nutritious yet low in calories, sugar, and saturated fat.
▸ Readily available in most markets.
▸ Easy to prepare and cost-effective.

The first requirement will come as no surprise; nutritiously rich foods that are low in calories should be a part of every healthy eating plan. But exactly how do foods qualify as nutrient-dense? They must contain a high amount of micronutrients (vitamins, minerals, and amino acids), be low in sugar (fewer than 5 grams per serving), and have proven qual-

ities that reduce the likelihood of chronic diseases and illness.[7] All of the foods that I have chosen are also fresh, whole foods. For the sake of convenience, I have included a few frozen-meal options for times when you're really in a pinch. Even with the best intentions and planning, life circumstances always seem to complicate our daily routines, and we don't always have time to prepare a meal from scratch. The frozen meals I have chosen are nutritious and contain very few (if any) preservatives or added sodium.

The second and third requirements aren't typically considered in most weight-loss programs. I focused on the cost and availability of foods when constructing my Core Envy Diet because I want the foods you're eating to be easy to find and easy on your wallet. In my 15 years of guiding people through weight-loss journeys, I've heard every excuse in the book about why it's impossible to follow the plan. Convenience and cost are the most common and legitimate complaints. If you've ever tried to follow a program that asks you to purchase Chinese cabbage and free-range elk tenderloins, you know exactly what I'm talking about. Convenience and cost determine the likelihood of your adherence to the plan.

Once I had my list of highly nutritious and low-calorie foods, I compared it to the USDA's list of food availability and the cost index for each item.[9] My goal was to give you a list of foods that are good for you while also being easy to find and cost-effective. For example, blackberries rank at the top of the list in terms of nutrient density, but they also rank very high in price (almost twice the price of blueberries) and can be difficult to find out of season. For this reason, you will see blueberries make the list but not blackberries.

Other foods that ranked high in nutrient density but didn't make the cut for cost and availability are guava, endive, beet greens, elk, and macadamia nuts. If you want to include these foods in your diet, please go ahead! Just make sure you are looking up the calorie content and tracking it in your food journal so that your daily calorie intake stays in check.

Can too much sodium really
AFFECT YOUR WAISTLINE?

We are told on a regular basis that we need to cut back on extra sodium in order to avoid high blood pressure, but the dangers of a high-sodium diet reach far beyond this one health concern. Studies show a direct correlation between high-sodium diets and the presence of elevated cortisol levels; remember that high cortisol levels create a cascade effect that triggers the body to store visceral abdominal fat around the organs (page 34). In addition, high-sodium diets have been directly linked to a greater risk of metabolic syndrome.[8] The recommended daily intake for sodium is 1,500 mg, or three-quarters of a tablespoon of table salt.

The Core Envy Diet is naturally low in sodium, but here is a short list of healthy foods that contain unusually high levels of sodium. Eat these foods in moderation:

▶ Shellfish (especially shrimp)

▶ Smoked meats and fish

▶ Deli meats

▶ Soy sauce, fish sauce, teriyaki sauce, and most other dark sauces

▶ Packaged soups

CORE ENVY FOODS

VEGETABLES

Asparagus

Broccoli

Brussels sprouts

Cabbage

Carrots

Cauliflower

Leafy greens: kale, spinach, arugula, collard greens, chard, etc.

Peas

Peppers: red, yellow, orange

Tomatoes, fresh

FRUITS

Apples

Bananas

Blueberries

Grapefruit

Oranges

Strawberries

PROTEIN*

Beef (at least 90% lean)

Chicken breast

Eggs

Seafood: cod, salmon, tuna

Shellfish: clams, oysters, crab

Turkey breast (no added nitrates)

*Organic, free-range/wild-caught

FATS

Almonds

Avocado

Olive oil

Peanuts

Pistachios

Sunflower seeds

GRAINS & CARBOHYDRATES

Brown rice

Oats

Polenta

Quinoa

Squash

Sweet potatoes/yams

LEGUMES

Black beans

Chickpeas/garbanzo beans

Lentils

Pinto beans

Tofu

TREAT YOUR BODY TO A DIET MAKEOVER

It will come as no surprise that the foods that consistently rank the highest in terms of being "good for you" are all fruits and vegetables. Despite all the research showing the fat-fighting, illness-depleting benefits of fruits and veggies, American consumption of these two food categories is far below the recommended amount. Instead, we consume more than the recommended amounts of fatty animal products and refined grains, both of which contribute to our ever-expanding waistlines.

Cut Out Refined Grains and Gluten

When it comes to grains, the American diet focuses predominantly on wheat. As of 2010, the per capita annual consumption of wheat was at an astounding 137 pounds. Unfortunately, almost all of those 137 pounds are finding their way onto our plates in refined and processed forms. Current data shows that only 7 percent of Americans are getting the recommended amount of whole grains, yet we are still consuming more total grains than recommended; on average we eat 6.68 ounces of grains per day, and 5.61 of those ounces are refined.[10]

Refined grains can contribute to unwanted weight gain because the process of stripping the bran and germ from the grain also strips away the fiber, which in turn causes the body to digest the grain quickly and also makes insulin spike. If your body is digesting food quickly, then you are prone to eat more calories than necessary because you don't feel full. As a reaction to all these extra calories, your body releases too much insulin and your

WHERE OUR DIETS FALL SHORT

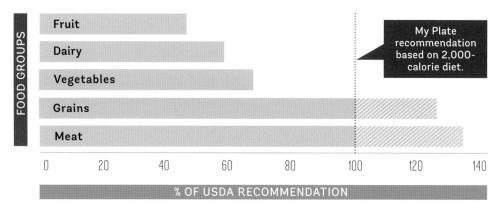

DECODING GRAINS

Labeling can be blamed for many of our poor decisions around whole grains. A loaf of bread that is labeled "whole grain" may only contain 1 percent whole grain and 99 percent refined grains. And just because something is labeled "wheat bread" doesn't mean that it contains whole-grain wheat—it is most likely wheat that is processed and refined, stripped of its nutritional benefits and loaded with additional sugar and preservatives.

To make better-informed choices when it comes to eating whole grains, you need to be able to decode the terminology found on the packaging so you can choose the grains that are highly nutritious and more conducive to maintaining an enviable core.

Whole grains. The term "whole" in the context of grains means that the entire kernel is used and nothing is stripped or taken away. A whole kernel of grain consists of three parts—the endosperm, germ, and bran.

Refined grains. Refining a grain entails taking away portions of the original kernel. In almost every case this means that the bran and germ are removed, oftentimes through techniques such as bleaching and bromating.

Enriched grains. If a grain is enriched, that means that something is added to it, which also implies that something has first been taken away. Often a grain is first refined (bran and germ removed) and then "enriched" by adding back nutrients that have been taken away, such as fiber, iron, and folic acid. Many times the nutrients that are added back are not in the same form; for example, metallic iron can be used as a substitute for naturally existing iron. Furthermore, added nutrients commonly represent a fraction of what the original grain contained.

Fortified grains. A fortified grain is one that has nutrients added to it that may or may not have existed in the original grain. One of the biggest criticisms of fortified foods is that the added nutrients are often more difficult for the body to absorb.

continues

DECODING GRAINS *continued*

With all these different terms being thrown around, how are we supposed to know which grains are healthy? One of the easiest ways to identify which foods contain whole grains is to look for the Whole Grain stamp that has been issued by the Whole Grains Council.

The "Basic Stamp" is used for foods that contain some whole grains, but not 100 percent of the grains used in the product are whole grain. The "100% Stamp" indicates that grains used in the product are 100 percent whole. Look for the 100% Stamp as often as possible, though products that have the Basic Stamp are also a good place to start. Some foods that are naturally whole grain will not carry the whole-grain stamp. The following grains and grasses are naturally whole grain.

NATURALLY WHOLE-GRAIN OPTIONS

Amaranth	Polenta
Brown rice	Quinoa
Buckwheat	Sorghum
Millet	Teff
Oats	Wild rice

blood sugar starts to take a roller-coaster ride. Scientists at the Harvard School for Public Health state that "easily digested refined carbohydrates . . . may contribute to weight gain, interfere with weight loss, and promote diabetes and heart disease."[11]

In addition to eliminating refined carbohydrates, if you can commit to cutting gluten out of your diet for the 8 weeks it takes to complete the Core Envy program, you will jump-start your weight loss. All of the grains found on my list are whole grains, and they all happen to be gluten-free. With gluten-free cookbooks and products flooding the market, you might be tempted to think my Core Envy Nutrition Plan is just a reflection of dietary groupthink. The truth is that cutting gluten out of your diet is an effective, efficient way to slim your waistline, get rid of bloating, and decrease sugar cravings.

Wheat, barley, and rye are the three grains that include gluten. While you are on the Core Envy program, simply switch out these grains for brown rice, oats, quinoa, and wild rice. I specifically choose these grains to be included in the list of foods because they are readily available in all markets and affordable. If there are other gluten-free whole grains that you enjoy eating, please feel free to include them in your diet. And once you are finished with the program, you can reintroduce gluten in the form of highly nutritious whole grains as part of a well-balanced diet.

Eat More Vegetables

For the Core Envy Diet to work, you will need to eat more vegetables. For most of us, this is the single biggest lifestyle change. There are many excuses for avoiding vegetables, but the most common form of resistance I find in clients (besides the statement that they are gross!) is that vegetables are expensive. Though this perception is widespread, the reality is that most vegetables are not only economical but easily accessible. According to a USDA report, we can get the recommended amount of vegetables and fruits for as little as $2 a day. To put this into perspective, the cost of that daily Starbucks coffee (not even the fancy drinks—just the regular drip coffee) is enough to cover your daily vegetable intake. Take the time to sit back and evaluate your finances when it comes to your food choices. My guess is that your pocketbook actually will

The beauty of a SHORTER SHOPPING LIST

You might look at the list of Core Envy foods and think it looks restrictive. What if you want to eat something that's not on the list? While it might seem difficult to focus your diet on a short list of foods, keep in mind that having too many options often leads to poor decisions. Over the years, I have approached weight-loss plans with my clients in every way possible: letting them choose their own foods, giving them new meal plans every week, and keeping them on a plan that is slightly repetitive yet consistent. Far and away the most successful plans have been the ones that keep my clients on a regular, consistent schedule that allows them to create a routine. Establishing healthy choices around food means staying focused on a short list that gives you the most bang for your buck, which is exactly what the foods list does for you.

PRODUCE BUYING GUIDE

DIRTY DOZEN (buy these organic)

Celery	Blueberries	Kale
Peaches	Nectarines	Cherries
Strawberries	Bell peppers	Potatoes
Apples	Spinach	Grapes (imported)

CLEAN 15 (lowest in pesticides)

Onions	Sweet peas	Cantaloupe
Avocado	Asparagus	Watermelon
Sweet corn	Kiwi	Grapefruit
Pineapple	Cabbage	Sweet potato
Mango	Eggplant	Honeydew melon

allow you to eat healthier, though it may require you to give up some of your go-to foods and drinks that aren't providing you with anything but convenience, extra calories, and the comfort of routine.

Organic options are always preferable when buying produce, but if your budget is tight, you can focus your organic purchases on the produce that tends to carry the highest concentration of pesticides when they are grown conventionally.

....

Now that you are armed with the knowledge of how different foods can affect your waistline, it's time to put the plan in place. Beginning on page 141, I will explain the nuts and bolts of how to implement your food plan. I've created meal plans, recipes, and food logs to help guide you. You might find that you prefer keeping track of your food with one of the myriad smart-phone apps that are available today, or, if you're like me, you might carry a little notebook in your purse so that you're forced to actually put pen to paper and write down those three snack-sized Snickers that magically appeared in your desk drawer. Regardless of how you choose to approach your Core Envy diet, visit www.coreenvybook.com to share recipes and get tips from others in the Core Envy community.

Eating healthy when you have no time, no creativity, and no cooking skills

I'M ONE OF THOSE LIFELONG DIETERS who has tried every plan in the book, and the reason nothing has ever worked for me is simple: I don't cook. By saying this, I mean it's a miracle if I assemble a sandwich. I've tried to become interested in cooking, but after years of stocking my refrigerator with mounds of fresh veggies and meats—only to watch 75 percent of the food go to waste as it sat there unused and rotting—I finally had to face the reality that I don't cook and I'm never going to start. My lack of interest in the kitchen has always been my biggest downfall with losing weight and keeping it off. It's 8 p.m., I'm tired and hungry, I have no food in the house, and a quick trip to the Mexican restaurant down the street suddenly seems like a great idea.

The Core Envy Diet has essentially solved all of my cooking woes. Not only are most of the suggested options available in restaurants and as ready-made meals at grocery stores but there are even guidelines for how to choose healthy frozen meals. This is a plan that actually works for a real person! I've even learned that I can get hard-boiled eggs in large quantities at places like Costco and that always having healthy bars on hand saves me from making poor snacking decisions. I also really like having a list of 40 foods to focus on. At this point I have the list memorized, and it takes all the guesswork out of my decisions around food. The fact that all 40 foods are easy to find and budget-conscious are two more reasons why this plan is realistic and sustainable. Finally, a weight-loss plan that fits my lifestyle!

the
CORE ENVY
PROGRAM

CORE ENVY
SCULPTING
exercises

NOW THAT WE KNOW how to go about tightening up your core, it's time to get to work! In this chapter you will find 30 different exercises, each of which has an easy, a moderate, and a challenging variation to accommodate your current physical ability. You can choose the level that best suits your overall skill. Because we all have different muscular imbalances and strengths, I encourage you to select the appropriate level for each individual exercise rather than simply doing, for example, Level 2 through all three routines. With 90 different movements comprised of three specific categories of movement—Balance & Isometrics, Pushing & Pulling, and Twisting & Bending—the Core Envy program works all of the muscles of your midsection to build a strong, sexy core.

Too often when we embark on a mission to improve our core strength, we do so in a cavalier, haphazard manner that is a mishmash of exercises we've learned over the years. The biggest mistake you can make with a core routine is to resort to the path of least resistance by doing crunches. Not only does this strengthen muscles that are already strong, it also exacerbates the strength discrepancy between the front and back sides of the core, and it can actually end up making your posture worse. In order to create an organized, scientifically sound method to work all the core muscles without neglecting or overworking any particular area, I've created a sculpting program that includes three different types of exercises. Each of these routines serves a different purpose in terms of sculpting, muscle activation, and strength.

Balance & Isometrics. Develops your ability to engage the deep muscles of the core so you'll get more out of all of your sculpting routines.

Pushing & Pulling. Works all of the muscles connected to the pelvis and spine to create stability as you move in the frontal plane (forward and backward).

Twisting & Bending. Works the rotational muscles of your core to build dynamic strength.

All of the sculpting exercises in my program have two things in common: They don't require a gym membership (take it on the road!), and they give equal attention to all the muscles in the core.

BALANCE & ISOMETRICS

These movements are foundational to establishing lasting, functional core strength. The exercises in this category focus on getting the muscles of the core that tend to be the laziest to wake up and start doing some work. Almost every exercise requires you to hold a specific pose for a designated amount of time (this is what makes it isometric), which can be challenging and a bit frustrating. You need to remain focused on the quality of your form during these routines, so don't zone out! Developing your ability to engage the deep muscles of the core is essential to completing the more complex exercises in the other routines.

PLANK HOLD

CORE FOCUS | all the muscles from your shoulders to the bottom of your hips

LEVEL 1

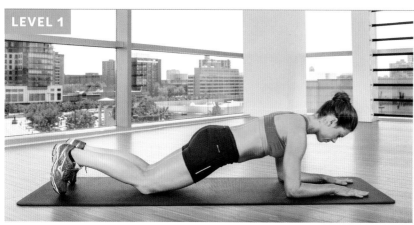

LEVEL 2

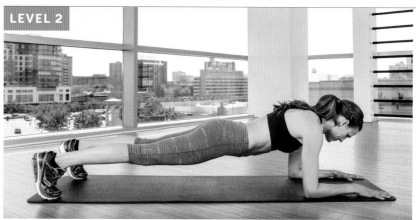

LEVEL 3

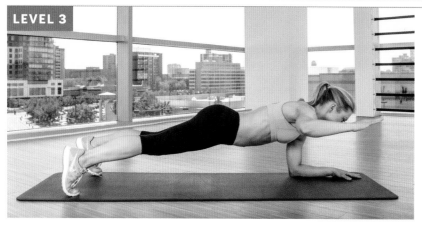

It's no coincidence that we begin our core strength routine with one of the most iconic of core exercises: the plank. By positioning your body parallel to the ground, you are removing the benefit of gravity in supporting your body weight. Instead, your core muscles must support the weight of your body.

ON YOUR KNEES

▸ **Hold 20–30 seconds to complete 1 set**

Lie facedown on the floor. Place your forearms parallel to each other, like a sphinx. Keeping your neck neutral (don't look up or down), push up onto your forearms and lift your chest. Keep your knees on the floor but actively engage your abdominals and glutes to hold your body in alignment. Think of gently puffing your low back up toward the ceiling while dropping your tailbone toward the floor. This should be a subtle, natural movement. Continue to breathe while holding this position.

ON YOUR TOES

▸ **Hold 30–45 seconds to complete 1 set**

Place your forearms parallel to each other on the floor. Push up onto your forearms and lift your chest. Actively engage your abdominals and glutes to hold the position. Be sure to keep your neck neutral and your ears in line with your shoulders, continuing to breathe as you hold this position. You might find yourself tempted to rock backward and lift your hips toward the ceiling as you fatigue. Fight to keep those hips low, shoulders directly over the hands, and tailbone slightly tucked!

WITH ELBOW RAISE

▸ **1 set is 10 repetitions on each side**

This version of the plank hold still focuses on an isometric hold in the trunk, but the arms will slowly lift out to the side to challenge that hold. Start in the basic plank position, then slowly raise one elbow out to the side, stopping when your elbow reaches shoulder height. Bring your forearm back down to the floor, then lift the opposite arm. Continue alternating arms to complete the set.

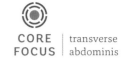

CORE FOCUS | transverse abdominis

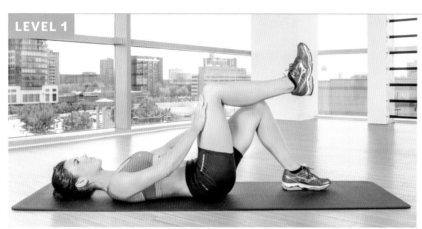

LEVEL 1

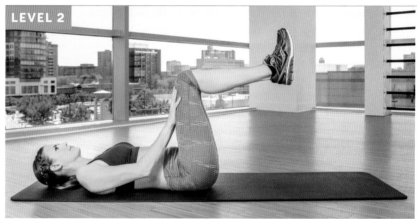

LEVEL 2

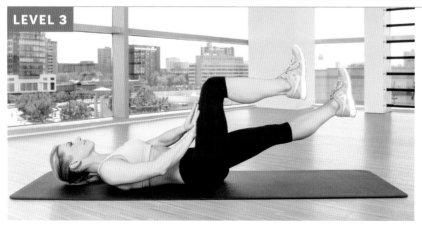

LEVEL 3

The transverse abdominis (TVA) is the deepest of the abdominal muscles, and most of us don't put it to good use. A strong and well-functioning TVA will improve posture, support your low back, and increase power output to your limbs. The first step to building a strong TVA is learning how to activate it on command. This exercise will help you make that mind-muscle connection.

ONE FOOT ON THE FLOOR ▸ **1 set is three 6-second repetitions on each leg**

Lie on your back with your head resting on the floor, knees bent, and both feet on the ground approximately 12 inches from your glutes. Raise one leg so that your knee makes a 90-degree angle, with your shin parallel to the floor. Keep your knee directly over your hip joint—do not bring it closer to your chest because this activates the rectus abdominis muscle, and we want that muscle to remain as relaxed as possible during this exercise. Place both hands on your thigh and gently push your hands into your thigh while resisting the push with your leg. This is an isometric contraction, so you shouldn't see your leg move. Push for 6 seconds, then rest for 6 seconds. After completing the set, switch to the other leg.

BOTH FEET LIFTED ▸ **1 set is four 6-second repetitions**

Lie on your back with your head resting on the floor and lift both legs to a 90-degree angle with your shins parallel to the ground. Keep your knees directly over your hips. Place one hand on each thigh and isometrically push against both legs at the same time. You are creating your own resistance here, so make sure you're resisting that push as hard as possible! Push for 6 seconds, then rest for 6 seconds.

ONE LEG EXTENDED ▸ **1 set is four 6-second repetitions on each leg**

Begin by lying on your back with both legs positioned at a 90-degree angle, then extend one leg out straight and place both hands on the thigh of the bent leg. Push for 6 seconds, then rest for 6 seconds, and complete the set before switching legs. As the movement becomes more challenging, remember to keep your head relaxed on the floor.

3 | SIDE PLANK

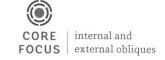
LEVEL 1

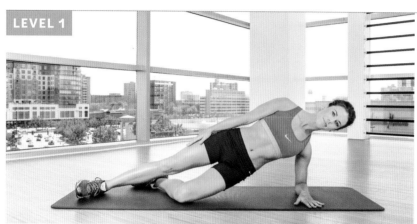

LEVEL 2

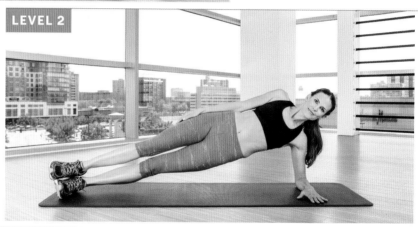

LEVEL 3

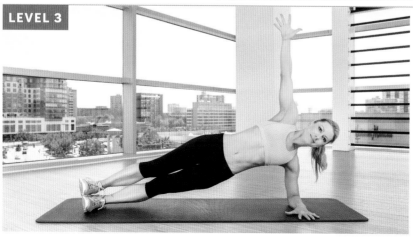

Side planks are a must-have exercise when it comes to strengthening the core because they recruit so many muscle fibers. This one is tough but well worth it!

WITH KNEE SUPPORT   ▸ Hold 20–30 seconds on each side to complete 1 set

Begin by lying on one side with your elbow positioned on the floor directly below your shoulder. Bend your bottom leg for stability and extend your top leg out straight. You can keep your top hand on the ground in front of your chest for extra support if you need it, but the goal is to rest your arm on your side or hip so you can engage more of your core muscles. Push down through your bottom elbow and lift your hips as high as possible from the floor. Your bottom knee will remain on the ground. Hold that position for 20 to 30 seconds and repeat on the opposite side.

WITHOUT SUPPORT   ▸ Hold 30–45 seconds on each side to complete 1 set

Start on your side with your elbow lined up beneath your shoulder and extend both legs out straight. Rest your top arm along your side and push down through your bottom elbow and forearm as you lift your hips high. Check to make sure that your body makes a straight line from your shoulders all the way down to your ankles.

WITH REACH   ▸ Hold 45–60 seconds on each side to complete 1 set

Get into side plank position with your elbow positioned below your shoulder and both legs extended. Push into the floor with your bottom elbow and forearm and lift your hips to make a straight line from your shoulders to your ankles. Reach your top hand toward the ceiling and hold steady to complete the set before repeating on the other side.

SINGLE-LEG BALANCE

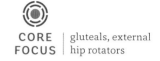

CORE FOCUS | gluteals, external hip rotators

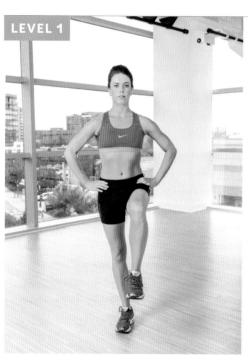

LEVEL 1

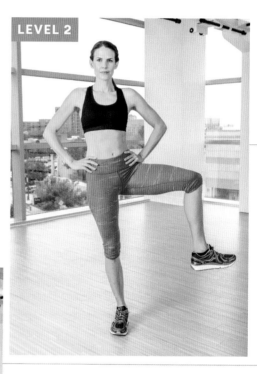

LEVEL 2

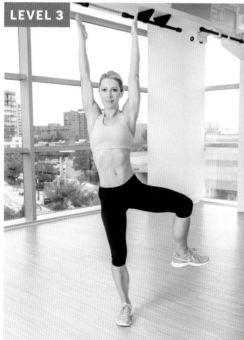

LEVEL 3

What is a single-leg exercise doing in a core routine? It improves the stabilization of the pelvis. When you lift one leg off the ground, the pelvis naturally shifts toward the standing leg in order to stack as much weight as possible over that leg. By engaging the glute on the standing leg, you will feel more stable and secure. If your balance is a little wobbly, try doing this exercise next to a countertop or stable surface that you can use for balance if needed.

WITH KNEE FORWARD ▸ Hold 20–30 seconds on each leg to complete 1 set

Stand with your feet slightly closer than hip-width apart, hands resting gently on your hips. Transfer all of your weight onto one foot and slowly lift the opposite foot off the floor. Squeeze the glutes on the standing leg and work toward getting the lifted leg to a 90-degree angle, with your knee level with your hip.

WITH KNEE OUT   ▸ Hold 30–45 seconds on each leg to complete 1 set

Stand with your feet slightly closer than hip-width apart and hands on your hips. Lift one leg to a 90-degree angle, then slowly swing it out to the side and hold it there. If tightness in the hips keeps you from lifting to the full 90-degree angle, lift as far as you can and eventually work toward a higher angle. Keep both hips steady and pointing forward as you hold this position.

WITH ARMS EXTENDED ▸ Hold 45–60 seconds on each leg to complete 1 set

Stand with your feet slightly closer than hip-width apart. Slowly swing one knee out to the side and hold it there. Raise your arms overhead, palms facing each other. Really engage the glutes on your standing leg to maintain your balance.

5 | WALL SIT

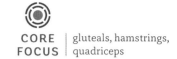

CORE FOCUS | gluteals, hamstrings, quadriceps

LEVEL 1

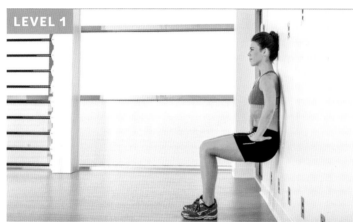

LEVEL 2

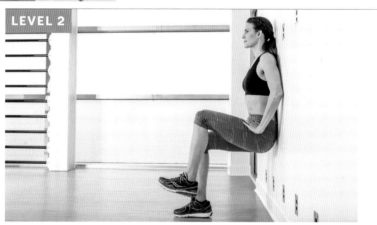

LEVEL 3

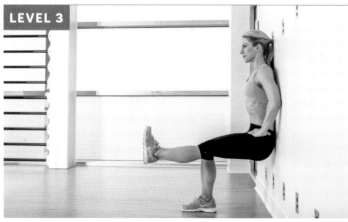

Here's another example of an exercise that doesn't seem as if it works the core. But remember that the quads, hamstrings, and gluteals are all part of the core because they are attached to the pelvis. Furthermore, the muscles surrounding the spine also have to work isometrically to maintain good posture in your upper body.

WITH BOTH FEET   ▸ Hold 30–60 seconds to complete 1 set

Stand with your back against a wall, feet shoulder-width apart. Walk your feet out to about 2 feet from the wall and slowly slide your back down the wall. Come as low as possible but no lower than a 90-degree angle at the knees. Keep the back of your head, shoulder blades, and glutes in contact with the wall at all times. Ideally your low back will be in contact with the wall as well, but you might have to work toward this as you gain strength in the deep core muscles.

WITH ALTERNATING FEET   ▸ 1 set is three 10-second holds on each leg

Slowly sink into a wall sit, keeping your head, shoulder blades, and glutes in contact with the wall. Raise one foot 6 inches off the floor and hold it for 10 seconds. Gently set that foot down and raise the opposite foot for 10 seconds. Continue alternating feet until you complete the set. Concentrate on gently pushing the full length of your spine against the wall the entire time.

WITH LEG EXTENDED   ▸ 1 set is five 10-second holds on each leg

Start in a squat position with your back against the wall. Try to bring your thigh bones parallel to the ground, though you may need to raise up a few inches until you build more strength. Pushing the entire length of your spine against the wall, contract your quadriceps muscles and extend one leg out straight. Hold this for as long as possible. If it's too challenging at first, begin by holding 2–3 seconds and build your stamina.

6 LUNGE

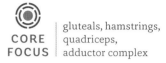

CORE FOCUS | gluteals, hamstrings, quadriceps, adductor complex

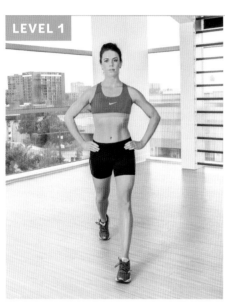

LEVEL 1

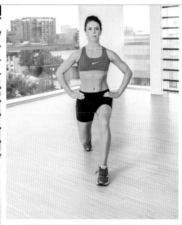

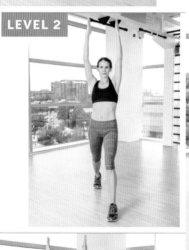

LEVEL 2

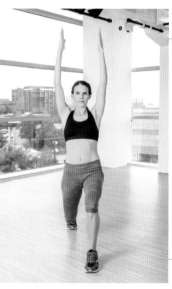

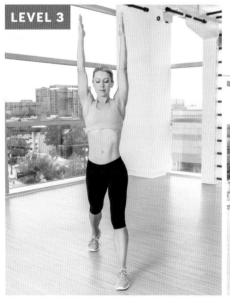

LEVEL 3

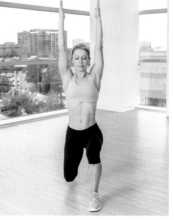

Just like the single-leg balance, lunges call upon the muscles of the core to help maintain proper alignment in the upper body and keep the body from tipping over. The first few times you try this exercise, stand next to a table or chair so that you can stabilize yourself if necessary.

HANDS ON HIPS ▸ 1 set is 10 repetitions on each leg

Step one foot forward into a long stance—there will be approximately 3–4 feet distance between your forward heel and the toes of your back foot. Keep your feet at least hip-width apart, or farther if you need additional help with balance. Squeeze your shoulder blades together, lift your chest, and align your ears over your shoulders. With your hands on your hips (or gently resting on a table or chair), lower your back knee toward the ground as if you're riding an elevator. Don't bend forward at the waist! If you have a history of knee pain, lower only as far as you can without pain. Lower and lift your back knee 10 times, then switch sides.

ARMS OVERHEAD ▸ 1 set is 12 repetitions on each leg

Step into a long stance with your feet positioned hip-width apart. Extend your arms straight up overhead, with palms facing each other. Your ears should be aligned with your shoulders. Keep your chest proud and shoulder blades together as you lower your body into the lunge. Go as low as you can while maintaining good alignment. Lower and lift 12 times, then switch sides.

ARMS OVERHEAD AND EYES CLOSED ▸ 1 set is 15 repetitions on each leg

Balance is more challenging with your eyes closed. Step into a long stance with your feet positioned hip-width apart. Extend your arms straight up overhead, palms facing each other. Align your ears with your arms and lower your shoulder blades toward your waistline. Close your eyes; you will immediately feel your balance become less secure. Tighten your core muscles and focus on a slow, controlled descent with your back knee. If you feel like you are going to tip over, open your eyes to regain your balance. Lower your back knee toward the ground and as you return to starting position, squeeze the glute on the back leg.

7

BIRD DOG

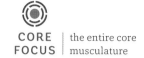

CORE FOCUS | the entire core musculature

LEVEL 1

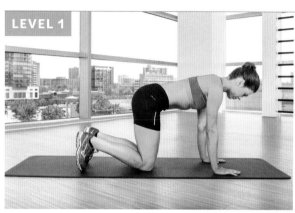

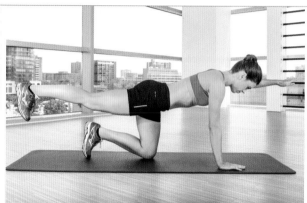

LEVEL 2

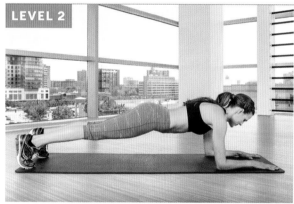

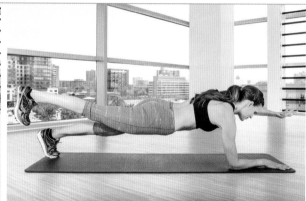

LEVEL 3

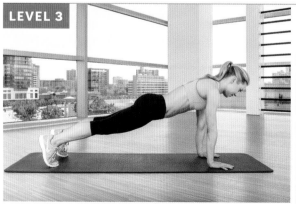

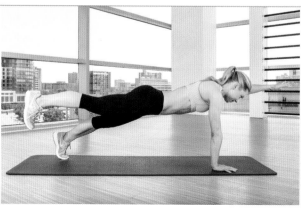

The bird dog gives the body practice in executing a cross-hemisphere movement, where the opposite hand and foot move in coordination with each other. This is one of those exercises that looks simple but is actually quite challenging. Don't rush through this—breathe with the movement and focus on the quality of the movement not the speed.

FROM QUADRUPED POSITION   ▶ **1 set is 10 repetitions on each side**

Begin in a quadruped position (on your hands and knees) with your hands directly below your shoulders and knees directly below your hips. Keeping your ears in line with your shoulders, reach one hand forward while you extend the opposite leg back. Keep your arm and leg parallel to the ground and think about trying to stretch the extension as much as possible. Hold for a few seconds, return to the starting position, and finish the repetitions before switching sides.

FROM PLANK ON FOREARMS   ▶ **1 set is 12 repetitions on each side**

Start in a forearm plank position with your elbows directly below your shoulders. Extend one arm forward and lift the opposite leg while keeping your hips up. Stretch the extension from your fingertips to your toes, remaining parallel to the ground. Hold this position for a few seconds before returning to the starting position. Do 12 extensions before switching sides. (If the plank position is too challenging, put your knees on the floor in modified plank position.)

FROM HIGH PLANK   ▶ **1 set is 15 repetitions on each side**

Start from a high plank or push-up position. Focus on squeezing the glutes while you lift one leg and extend the opposite arm forward. Hold it for a few seconds before lowering your arm and leg back into the starting position, working to lower the hand and foot to touch the ground at the same time. This exercise is more challenging, so try to slow down your breathing as you complete a set of 15 reaches, then switch sides.

8

BOAT POSE

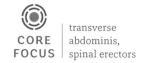

CORE
FOCUS | transverse
abdominis,
spinal erectors

LEVEL 1

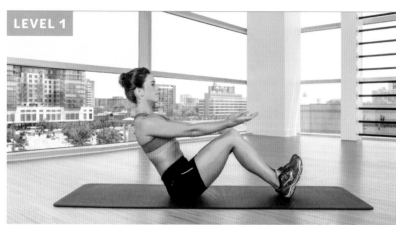

LEVEL 2

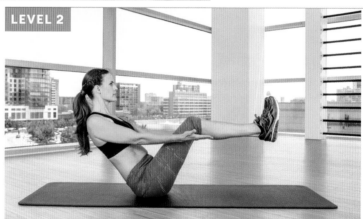

LEVEL 3

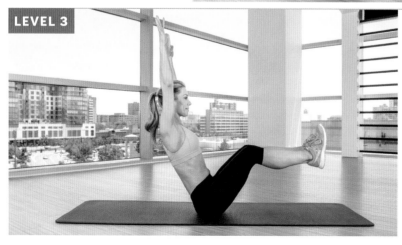

Boat pose is one of the iconic yoga poses that builds balance from a seated position. There are myriad variations, but for this routine we will focus on the isometric aspect.

WITH FEET ON FLOOR   ▸ Hold 20–30 seconds to complete 1 set

Begin in a seated position. Bend your knees and place your heels lightly on the floor, approximately 2 feet from your glutes. Elongate your spine, pull your shoulder blades down and back, and keep your neck neutral by gazing forward at the horizon. Extend your arms out straight in front of the body, parallel to the floor and palms open to the ceiling. Slowly begin to lean back until you feel a good shake in the core muscles. Maintain an elongated posture through the spine as you hold this position.

WITH FEET UP   ▸ Hold 30–45 seconds to complete 1 set

Lean back into boat pose from a seated position. Keep your spine long and neck neutral as you pull your shoulder blades down and back. Lift your heels until your shins are parallel to the floor. Extend your arms forward, palms facing the ceiling and arms parallel to the floor—hold this position.

WITH ARMS EXTENDED   ▸ Hold 45–60 seconds to complete 1 set

From a seated position, tip back onto your tailbone into boat pose. Keep your spine long and neck neutral as you pull your shoulder blades down and back. Lift your heels until your shins are parallel to the floor. Extend your arms overhead, palms facing forward. Remember to breathe normally as you hold this position.

9

SUPERMAN SERIES

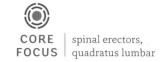

CORE FOCUS | spinal erectors, quadratus lumbar

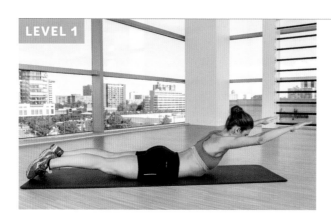

LEVEL 1

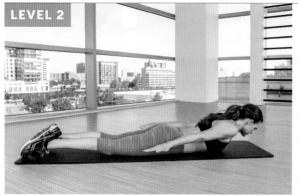

LEVEL 2

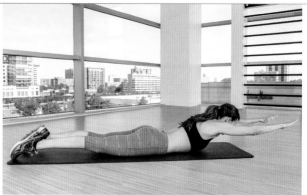

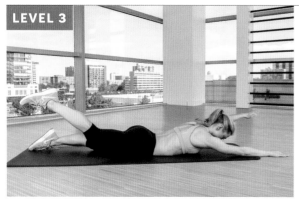

LEVEL 3

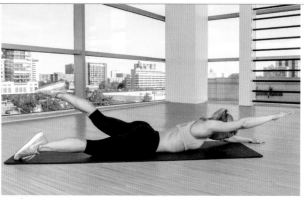

The muscles of the back are frequently neglected in our core training routines, though they are just as important as the muscles on the front side of the body in terms of establishing muscle tone, good posture, and functional strength.

UPPER BODY

▶ **Hold 10–15 seconds to complete 1 set**

Begin lying facedown on the floor or mat with your arms extended straight overhead. Keep the back of your neck long by looking down at the floor. Squeeze your glutes and raise your hands and chest off the ground, aiming to get your hands 6 inches off the floor. Hold this position.

UPPER BODY WITH ARM SWEEP

▶ **1 set is 12 repetitions**

Begin lying facedown on the floor or mat, arms extended down by your sides with palms facing the floor. Keeping the back of your neck long, squeeze your glutes and shoulder blades, raise your chest off the ground, and sweep your arms in a big arc until they are overhead. Bring your arms back down to starting position and relax your chest back to the floor between each repetition.

UPPER AND LOWER BODY ▶ **1 set is 15 repetitions on each side, alternating**

Lie facedown on the floor or mat with your arms extended in front of you, palms facing the floor. Raise one foot 6 inches off the ground and focus on squeezing the glute and extending the leg. At the same time, lift your chest and extend the opposite arm. Return to your starting position before reaching with the opposite leg and arm. Continue alternating sides until you complete the set.

10

HIGH PLANK SERIES

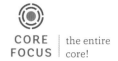

CORE FOCUS | the entire core!

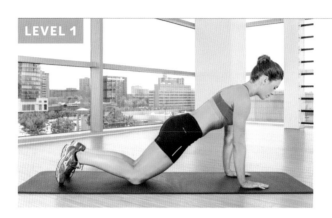

LEVEL 1

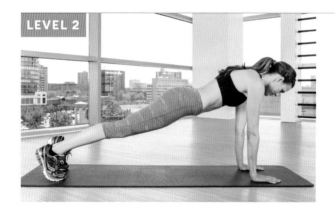

LEVEL 2

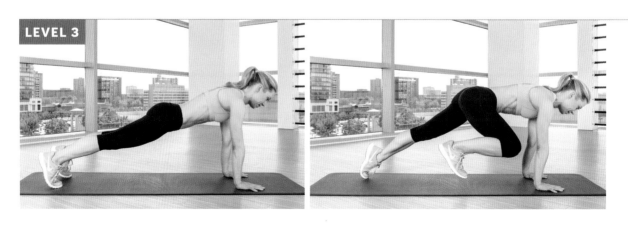

LEVEL 3

A high plank is essentially push-up position. It challenges the body a bit more than a forearm plank because you don't have the additional surface area to assist with balance. This is a building block for exercises in the other routines, so make it your goal to master it.

FROM KNEES

▶ **Hold 20–30 seconds to complete 1 set**

Come into a basic push-up position, but keep your knees on the ground. Keep your hands directly below your shoulders and engage the muscles in your core by actively pulling your belly button toward your spine. Keep your neck neutral by keeping your ears in line with your shoulders and hold this position.

FROM TOES

▶ **Hold 30–45 seconds to complete 1 set**

Start in push-up position with your hands positioned under your shoulders. Be sure to lift up through the upper back and slightly tuck your tailbone under to maintain a straight line from your shoulders to your ankles. Hold this position.

WITH KNEES DRIVING FORWARD

▶ **1 set is 15 repetitions with each leg**

Start in a high plank position with your hands directly below your shoulders and your core actively engaged. Slowly bring your right knee toward your right elbow, then back to starting position. Finish the repetitions before switching sides.

PUSHING & PULLING

All but one of the exercises in this routine require you to move with each repetition, as opposed to holding a stable position as you would for the balance and isometrics exercises. The only equipment you need is floor discs or a set of hand towels so that you can slide on the floor. If you are doing these exercises on carpet, try using paper plates or Frisbees.

Remember that the core consists of all muscles that are connected to the pelvis and spine, which means that the glutes and hamstrings are technically core muscles. That's why you will be doing squats and hip bridges in this routine. As your core strength improves and you're able to call upon the glutes and hamstrings, you will quickly realize how important they are to creating stability in the core when the rest of your body is moving!

1 PRONE COBRA

CORE FOCUS spinal erectors, quadratus lumbar, rhomboids, latissimus dorsi, lower trapezius

LEVEL 1

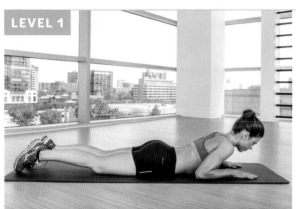

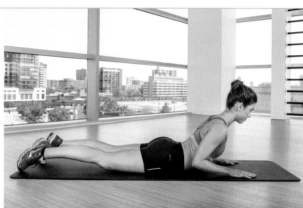

LEVEL 2

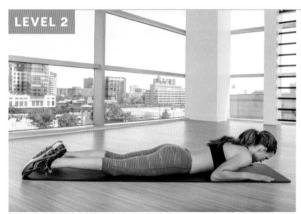

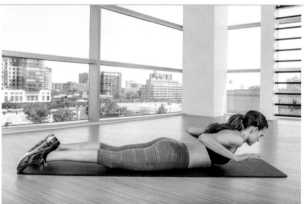

LEVEL 3

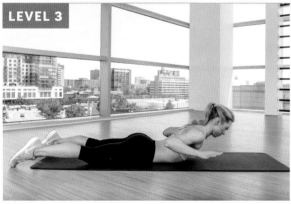

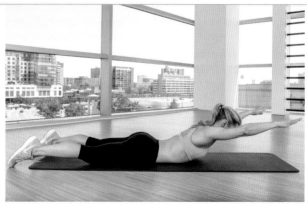

It's time to work the muscles of the back again! In the Balance & Isometrics routine, we focused on holding a back extension in an isometric position. In this section, we work on pushing and pulling the shoulder blades into different positions while the low back is in a gentle extension.

WITH ARMS PARALLEL

▸ **1 set is 10 repetitions**

Start in prone position with your forearms on the floor and parallel to each other. Gently squeeze your shoulder blades and begin to lift your chest off the ground, pushing your forearms into the floor. Keep the back of your neck long and your chin tucked. Once you reach the top of your range of motion, return to starting position.

WITH ARMS RAISED

▸ **1 set is 12 repetitions**

From a prone position, lift your forearms and gently begin to squeeze your shoulder blades together as you raise your upper body 6–8 inches off the floor. Return to starting position and repeat the movement until you have finished the set.

WITH ARMS EXTENDED

▸ **1 set is 15 repetitions**

Start in prone position with your forearms parallel to each other, held 6–8 inches from the floor. Squeeze your shoulder blades together as you lift your upper body into cobra position. When you get to the top of your range of motion, extend your arms straight out in front of you. If your shoulders feel tight, you might finish just short of full extension. Pull your elbows back down to your sides and keep your chest lifted off the floor as you finish the set.

2

SINGLE-LEG KICKS

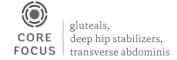

CORE FOCUS | gluteals, deep hip stabilizers, transverse abdominis

LEVEL 1

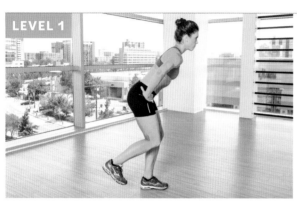

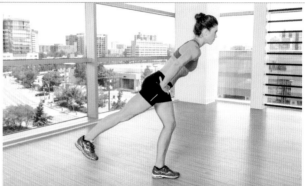

LEVEL 2

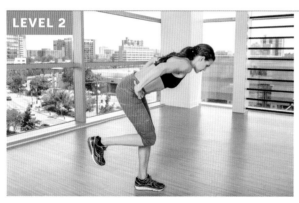

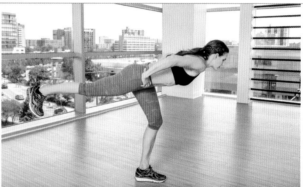

LEVEL 3

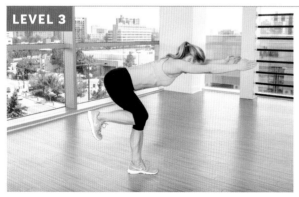

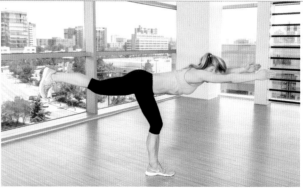

This is a hip extension exercise that works the gluteal muscles as well as the deep stabilizers of the hips. In this series we will also challenge the deep abdominal muscles by moving the upper body into different positions. Focus on tall posture as you do this exercise. It's a good idea to have a chair or table nearby in case you need a little extra support.

WITH FORWARD LEAN

▸ **1 set is 10 repetitions on each leg**

With hands on your hips (or gently resting on the back of a chair), lean slightly forward at the waist until your upper body is at a 45-degree angle with the floor. Slowly pick up one leg, keep your hips level, squeeze the gluteals of the lifted leg, and push your foot out behind your body. Concentrate on using the gluteal muscles to push—don't let the pelvis tip forward or the low back sink into an arch. Bring your leg forward to starting position and finish repetitions before switching sides.

WITH FORWARD BEND

▸ **1 set is 12 repetitions on each leg**

With hands on your hips, bend forward at the waist until your upper body is parallel with the floor. Keep your spine straight and tuck your chin so the back of your neck is long. Pull your belly button toward your spine and lift one foot off the ground. Gently squeeze your shoulder blades so that your upper back doesn't round, then extend your lifted leg out behind you. The goal is to create a "T" with your body. Bring the extended leg back under your body and then push it right back out. If this is too challenging, set your foot down for just a few seconds between repetitions. Finish repetitions before switching sides.

WITH ARMS EXTENDED

▸ **1 set is 15 repetitions on each leg**

Bend forward at the waist until your torso is parallel to the ground. Keeping your shoulder blades slightly squeezed, extend both arms forward so that your upper arms are in line with your head and parallel with the floor. Pick one foot up, engage the glutes on the working side, and extend your leg straight out behind you. Try to keep your arms extended and your torso parallel to the ground as you push and pull your leg out and in to complete the repetitions, then switch sides.

3

PUSH-UPS

CORE FOCUS | transverse abdominis, rectus abdominis, pectorals

LEVEL 1

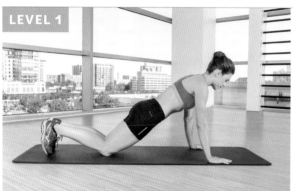
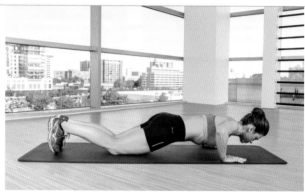

LEVEL 2

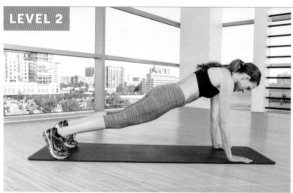
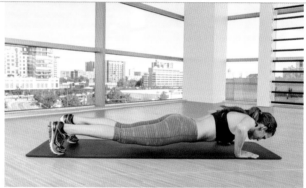

LEVEL 3

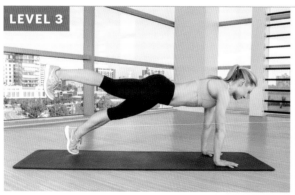
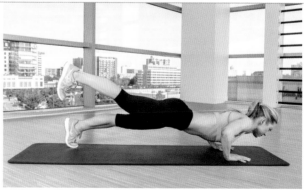

Here's an exercise that women (including me) love to hate, but this time-honored movement actually calls upon the core musculature as much as—if not more than—the upper body. As your core becomes stronger, you'll find that these muscles are able to assist in the movement as you progress through the levels.

FROM KNEES

▶ **1 set is 10 repetitions**

Start on your knees and place your hands on the floor directly below your shoulders. Gently drop your tailbone toward the floor and puff your low back out. Keeping the back of your neck long and your chin tucked, begin to bend your elbows into a 45-degree angle with your torso. Start by lowering your torso until your upper arms are parallel to the floor—if you're able to do this without your low back sagging or your hips moving out of alignment, then try bringing your chest even closer to the floor on the next repetition.

FROM TOES

▶ **1 set is 12 repetitions**

This is a traditional push-up in its finest form! Start in a push-up position, keeping your hands below your shoulders and your feet hip-width apart. It's common to want to push your hips backward so that your shoulders are behind your hands and your hips rise up toward the ceiling—avoid this because it places undue stress on the muscles around the rotator cuff. If you can't keep your hands directly below your shoulders and your hips low, do the Level 1 variation until you build more strength. As you lower your upper body to the floor, focus on keeping your hips stable; don't allow them to sag or to hike up toward the ceiling.

FROM SINGLE LEG

▶ **1 set is 8 repetitions on each leg**

Now it's time to incorporate balance and stability into your push-ups. Start in a traditional push-up position. Keep your feet wider than hip width in this variation in order to gain some additional balance. Slowly lift one foot off the ground, lower down into a push-up, and return to starting position. Try to keep that foot off the ground for all 8 repetitions, then switch sides.

CORE FOCUS | transverse abdominis, pectorals, rectus abdominis

LEVEL 1

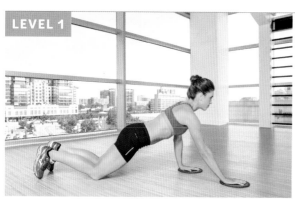

LEVEL 2

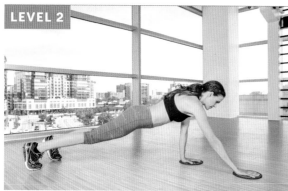

LEVEL 3

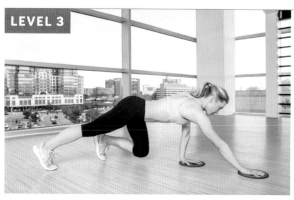

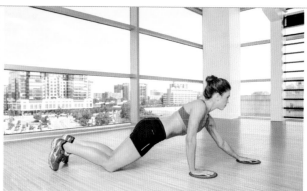

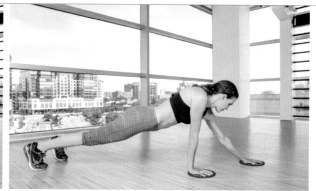

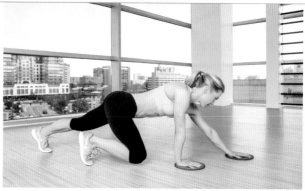

Learning to stabilize the torso while moving your limbs is an essential part of functional core strength. This exercise keeps the lower body stable (in Levels 1 and 2) while the upper arms glide forward and back. Level 3 experiments with upper- and lower-body coordination.

FROM KNEES

▸ **1 set is 10 repetitions on each side**

Begin on your knees in a push-up position with a glider or towel under each hand. Keep your torso long and don't let your hips droop or pop up toward the ceiling. Gently slide one hand forward about 6 inches. If you find that 6 inches is a little too intense, go as far as you can—even 2 inches will challenge the core. Move your hand back to the starting position and slide the opposite hand forward. Continue alternating sides until you finish the set.

FROM TOES

▸ **1 set is 12 repetitions on each side**

Get into push-up position with a glider or towel under each hand. Place your feet hip-width apart, or farther for more stability. The goal is to keep the hips even and parallel to the ground throughout the exercise. Slide one hand forward at least 6 inches. Slowly pull it back to starting position and slide your opposite hand forward. Alternate sides until you finish the set.

FROM TOES AND ARMS

▸ **1 set is 15 repetitions on each side**

Begin in a push-up position with a glider or towel under each hand. As you slide one arm forward, step forward with the opposite foot. Return to the starting position and repeat the motion with the opposite arm and foot. Be sure to keep the torso long during this movement and extend long through the front arm and back foot. Continue alternating sides until you complete the set.

5 JACKKNIVES

CORE
FOCUS | transverse abdominis,
iliopsoas, quadriceps,
gluteals

LEVEL 1

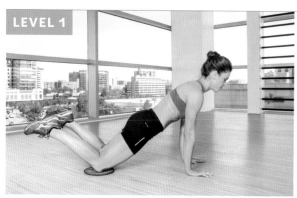

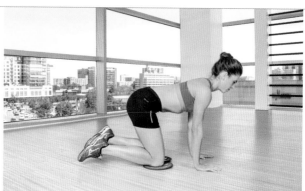

LEVEL 2

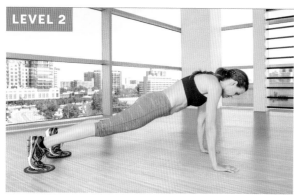

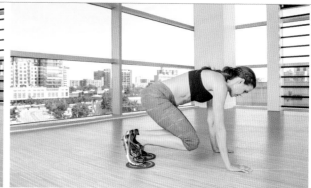

LEVEL 3

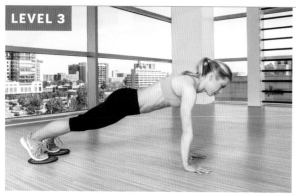

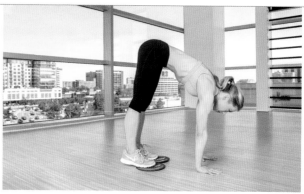

This is another movement that involves sliding, but this time you will keep the upper body stable while pushing and pulling the legs to work the core. I use this exercise with cyclists to teach the body how to effectively transfer energy from the core to the legs.

FROM KNEES

▸ **1 set is 10 repetitions**

Begin in a push-up position with your knees on the ground and a glider or towel under each knee. Keeping your core engaged and the back of your neck long, slowly pull both knees in toward your hands, then push them back to starting position. If you find that you feel "stuck" with your knees pulled in, you can push them back out one at a time.

FROM TOES TO TUCK

▸ **1 set is 12 repetitions**

Place a glider or towel under each foot and get into push-up position. Keeping your hands planted under your shoulders, bend your knees and slowly pull your feet in toward your hands. When you have brought your feet in as close as they can go comfortably, push them back out to starting position.

FROM TOES TO PIKE

▸ **1 set is 15 repetitions**

Begin in push-up position with a glider or towel under each foot. Keep your legs straight as you pull your feet in toward your hands and lift your hips up into a pike. When you have brought your feet as close to your hands as they can go comfortably, push them back out to starting position. Keep the movement smooth and controlled as you finish the set.

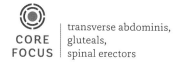

CORE FOCUS | transverse abdominis, gluteals, spinal erectors

LEVEL 1

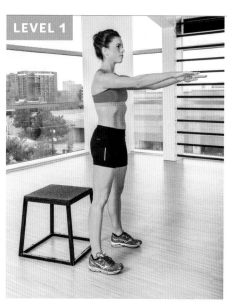

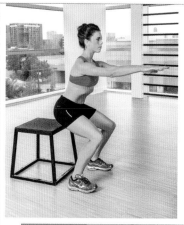

LEVEL 2

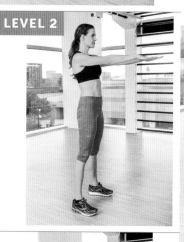

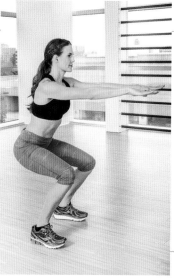

LEVEL 3

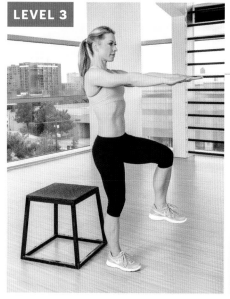

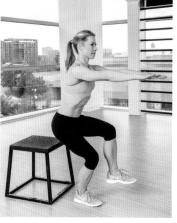

The squat might be the single most important movement for you to master. In a given day, you might perform some version of a squat between 50 and 100 times, depending on how often you stand up and sit down, get in and out of your car, and bend over to pick something up. If your core isn't strong enough to support your spinal column during a squat, you will end up rounding the shoulders and collapsing in the chest, which puts undue pressure on the low back.

WITH SUPPORT

▸ **1 set is 10 repetitions**

Stand in front of a chair with your feet hip-width apart. Lift your chest, pull your shoulder blades down and back, and gently engage your core by letting your tailbone drop downward. Shift your weight onto your heels (I actually lift up my toes inside my shoes) and push your hips back as far as possible. Try to keep your chest lifted and your knees behind your toes as you lower your hips to touch the chair. If you experience any pain in your low back or knees, come down only as far as you can without feeling pain. Squeeze your glutes and think of driving your hips forward as you return to standing position.

WITHOUT SUPPORT

▸ **1 set is 12 repetitions**

If you can execute a squat fluidly, take the chair away and let your body move freely through space. Stand with your feet hip-width apart. Keep your chest lifted and shoulder blades down and back; feel your weight in your heels as you lower down into squat position. Once your thighs are parallel to the floor, contract your glutes and drive your hips forward to reach the start position.

WITH A SINGLE LEG

▸ **1 set is 8 repetitions on each leg**

To do single-leg squats, begin with your feet hip-width apart, chest lifted, and shoulder blades pulled down and back. Shift your weight to one foot and lift the opposite foot off the floor. Feel your weight in the heel of the standing leg, push your hips back, and begin to lower into a squat. You will not be able to achieve a 90-degree angle; go only as far down as you can without letting the knee of the squatting leg move forward over your toes. Finish the repetitions before switching legs.

7 HIP BRIDGES

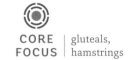

CORE FOCUS | gluteals, hamstrings

LEVEL 1

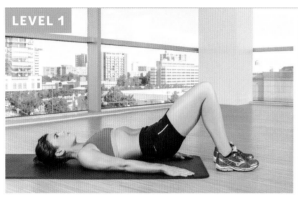 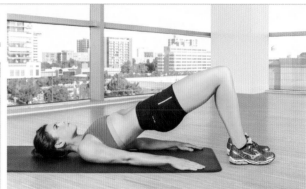

LEVEL 2

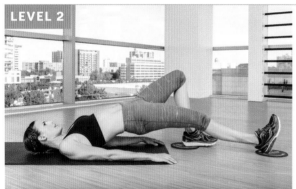 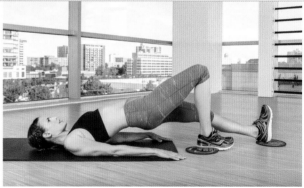

LEVEL 3

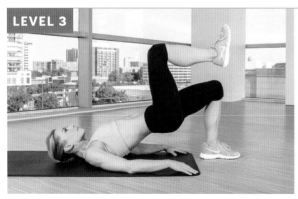 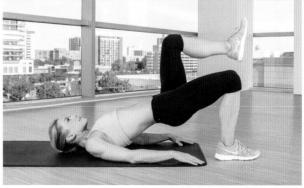

I love this exercise because it works the gluteals and the muscles on the back side of the core while being easy on the knees. It's quite common to feel the quadriceps attempting to do all the work during this movement, so try to focus on releasing the quads and forcing the glutes and hamstrings to fire.

WITH FEET TOGETHER ▸ **1 set is five 10-second repetitions**

Start on your back with your knees bent and feet on the floor approximately 12 inches away from your glutes. Relax your arms on the floor, palms down at your sides. Squeeze your glutes, tuck your tailbone, and lift your hips off the ground. Hold this position for 10 seconds, then lower your hips back down to the ground and rest for 5 seconds between repetitions.

WITH LEG EXTENSIONS ▸ **1 set is 12 repetitions on each side, alternating**

Lie on your back with your knees bent and a glider or towel under each foot. Keep your arms relaxed at your sides as you lift your hips off the floor. Slowly slide one foot away from your body until your leg is completely straight, then pull it back in. Repeat this pushing and pulling motion with the opposite foot. Keep your hips stable as you continue alternating sides.

WITH LEG LIFTS ▸ **1 set is 15 repetitions on each side, alternating**

Start in a basic hip bridge (on your back, hips in line with your shoulders and knees), and then lift your foot off the ground in a marching motion and slowly set it back down—no stomping! Alternate feet until you've completed the designated number of repetitions. Try to minimize any rocking in the hips. If you need to start with a smaller movement to stabilize the hips, lift your foot just 6 inches off the floor.

FROG LEGS

CORE FOCUS transverse abdominis, gluteals, abductor complex, hip external rotators

LEVEL 1

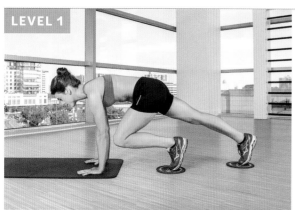
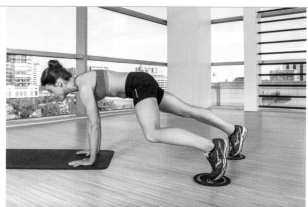

LEVEL 2

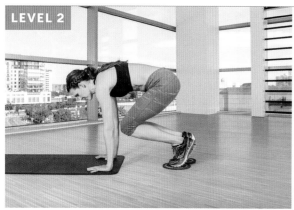
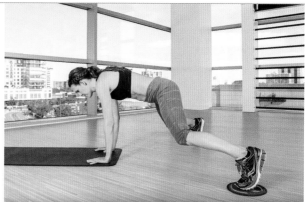

LEVEL 3

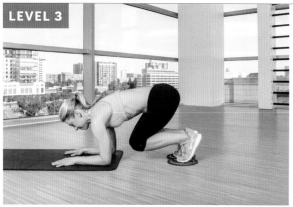
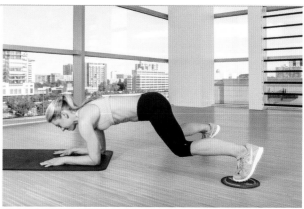

This exercise rounds out the triad that includes the sliding series and jackknives. The sliding series stabilized the core and lower body while moving the arms, and the jackknives stabilized the upper body while moving the legs forward and backward. With frog legs you will move your legs in a circle while holding both your core and upper body steady. If you have any experience doing the breaststroke in the pool, this exercise mimics the kicking portion of that stroke.

SINGLE-LEG MOTION

▸ **1 set is 10 repetitions on each side**

Begin in push-up position with your shoulders directly over your hands and a glider or towel under each foot. Keeping your core engaged, slowly pull your knee in toward your chest and then push it out in a circular motion before pulling it back into start position. Keep the supporting leg stationary throughout the exercise. This will provide stability for your lower back while you learn the movement. Complete 10 repetitions before switching sides.

BOTH LEGS IN MOTION

▸ **1 set is 12 repetitions**

Begin in push-up position with your shoulders directly over your hands and a glider or towel under each foot. Engage your core as you slowly pull your knees in toward your chest and then turn your toes out in a circular motion before sliding them back to start position. By moving both legs at the same time, you will need to recruit muscles throughout the core and upper body to remain stable.

FROM PLANK POSITION

▸ **1 set is 15 repetitions**

Let's get your chest a little closer to the ground for a bigger challenge! Complete the frog-kick motion from a plank position on your forearms. Engage your core as you pull your knees in toward your chest and then turn your toes out in a circular motion. Slide your feet in a wide arc, then smoothly pull them back to start position.

STRAIGHT-LEG DROPS

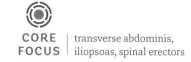

CORE FOCUS | transverse abdominis, iliopsoas, spinal erectors

LEVEL 1

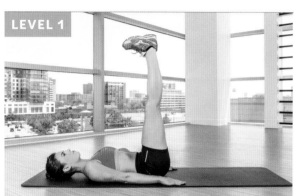
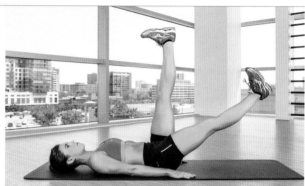

LEVEL 2

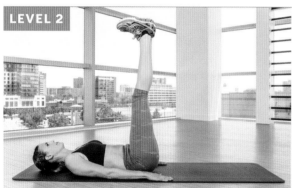
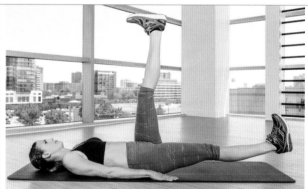

LEVEL 3

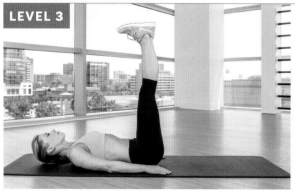
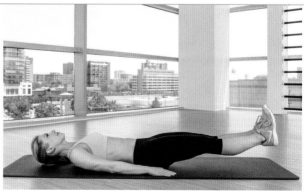

This exercise is a great way to practice controlled deceleration (the speed at which your muscles elongate). If you find that your lower back is arching during this movement, be sure to stick with Level 1 until you can successfully complete the next level while maintaining good form.

SPLIT, LIMITED RANGE OF MOTION ▸ 1 set is 10 repetitions with each leg

Begin on your back with both legs extended straight upward. Trying to keep your legs as straight as possible, pull your toes back toward your chest as if you were going to make a footprint on the ceiling. Keeping one leg straight, slowly lower the other leg halfway down toward the floor on a count of 2 seconds. Do not go farther down than 45 degrees. Slowly lift your leg back up to the starting position to a count of 2 seconds and repeat the movement, alternating legs.

FULL RANGE OF MOTION ▸ 1 set is 12 8-second repetitions with each leg

Now you are ready to lower your heel all the way to the ground and to spend a little more time doing it. Lie on your back and lower one leg at a time, slowing down the movement to take 4 seconds to lower and 4 seconds to lift, alternating legs.

LEGS TOGETHER ▸ 1 set is 15 8-second repetitions

Both legs are going down at the same time! Test the waters on this double-leg version by lowering halfway (to a count of 2 seconds) down. If you can complete this movement without pain or arching in the low back, then continue to get lower and lower toward the ground. Eventually you will lower both legs all the way to the ground to a count of 4 seconds and bring them back up to a count of 4.

CORE FOCUS | transverse abdominis, iliopsoas, spinal erectors, quadriceps

LEVEL 1

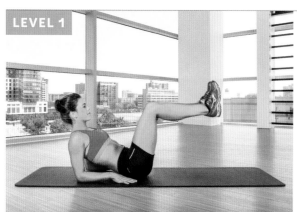

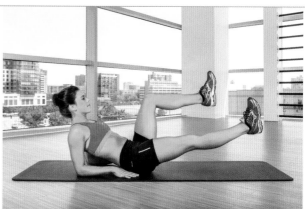

LEVEL 2

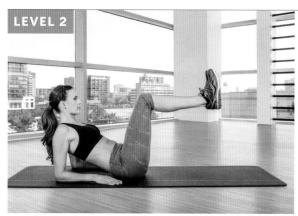

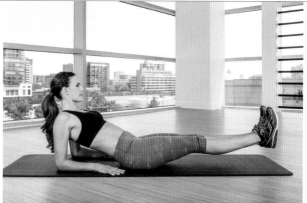

LEVEL 3

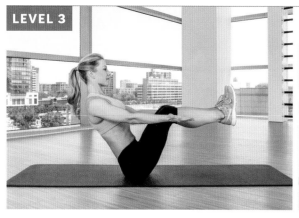

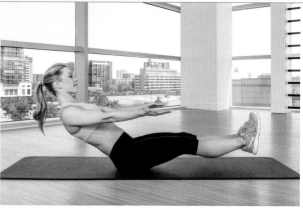

This exercise builds upon the isometric boat pose in Balance & Isometrics. You get to use that isometric strength while moving your legs in and out. Anytime the core musculature is asked to stabilize the pelvis while the legs move, there is a chance that your pelvis will rock forward and place strain on your low back. If you find this happening, simply back it down a level until you find the position that challenges the muscles of your low back but doesn't cause pain.

SINGLE-LEG EXTENSION ▸ 1 set is 10 repetitions with each leg, alternating

Begin by leaning back on your forearms, elbows positioned on the floor slightly behind your torso and fingertips pointing forward. As you lean back, keep your chest open and wide. With your knees bent, bring your legs up to form a 90-degree angle with the floor. Slowly extend one leg all the way out, bring it back to the starting position, then extend the opposite leg. Continue to alternate legs while keeping your upper body stable.

DOUBLE-LEG EXTENSION ▸ 1 set is 12 repetitions

Lean back on your forearms with your elbows stacked beneath your shoulders. Work to keep your tailbone tucked and don't allow the low back to arch or rock as you lift your heels off the floor. The deep stabilizing muscles around the pelvis will be challenged a bit more when you work both legs at the same time. Engage those muscles as you bring your knees in toward your chest, stopping when they are stacked over your hips and your shins are parallel to the floor. Pushing through your heels, extend your legs back to start position. If you need to modify this exercise, start by extending both legs halfway and work up to the full extension.

WITH ARMS EXTENDED ▸ 1 set is 15 repetitions

If you're a yoga practitioner, you may be familiar with this exercise, which is sometimes called high boat, low boat. Lean back, balancing your weight on your tailbone as you lift your legs, shins parallel to the floor. Extend your arms forward, palms open to the ceiling—this is the starting position. Keeping your shoulder blades pulled down and back and your chest open, lean back into low boat as you push your legs into extension. Pause here before returning to the starting position. Don't rush the movement.

TWISTING & BENDING

Now the fun really begins! In my experience, core exercises that require twisting and bending are most often ignored, mainly because it's difficult to come up with creative options that fit into this category. Not anymore! This Twisting & Bending routine will work the rotational muscles of the core in ways you have never experienced before. Because these movements ask the spine to rotate and bend, pay attention to any aches and pains that might arise. If you have chronic sciatic nerve pain, you should be especially careful with these exercises. Start at Level 1 and do the movements slowly and with intention.

1

TWISTING SIDE PLANK SERIES

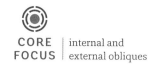

CORE FOCUS | internal and external obliques

LEVEL 1

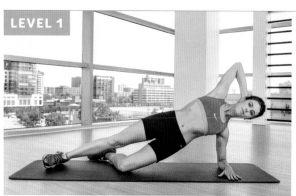 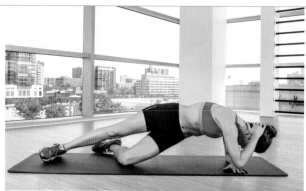

LEVEL 2

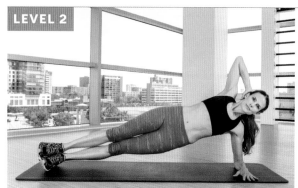 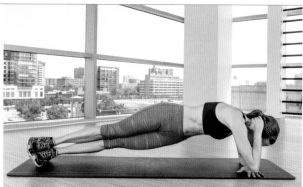

LEVEL 3

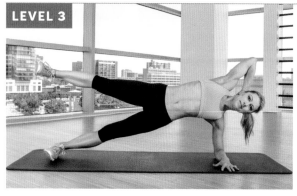 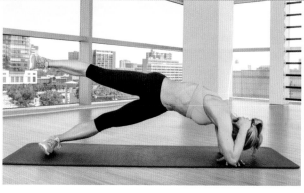

You were introduced to side planks in the Balance & Isometrics routine, where you learned how to set up the foundational pose and hold it for a given amount of time. In this exercise, you'll call upon the balance that you have developed and add to it an upper-body twist to create rotational strength through the core.

WITH KNEE ON THE FLOOR
▸ **1 set is 10 repetitions on each side**

Start on your side and position your forearm on the floor, keeping your elbow directly below your shoulder. Keep your top leg straight and bend the lower leg to form a 90-degree angle. Lift your hips to create a straight line from your top shoulder down to your ankle. The bottom knee remains on the floor throughout this exercise to provide support for the low back. Hold your hand behind your head so your elbow is pointing up at the ceiling. Twist your torso as you bring your elbow toward your stationary hand.

WITH BOTH LEGS STRAIGHT
▸ **1 set is 12 repetitions on each side**

Come into a side plank position with both legs extended out straight, feet stacked on top of each other. Check to make sure your body makes a straight line from your head all the way down to your feet. Lift your hips toward the ceiling and find your balance, then place your hand behind your head and twist your torso until your elbow reaches the floor.

WITH TOP LEG LIFTED
▸ **1 set is 15 repetitions on each side**

Come into a side plank position with legs extended and feet stacked on top of each other. Lift your hips toward the ceiling, bringing your body into alignment from your head all the way down to your feet. Hold your hand behind your head and lift your top leg, foot flexed. While keeping your leg lifted, twist your torso to touch your elbow to the supporting hand on the floor.

2

"C" SERIES

CORE FOCUS | internal and external obliques, iliopsoas

LEVEL 1

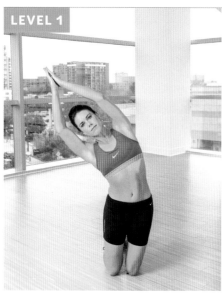

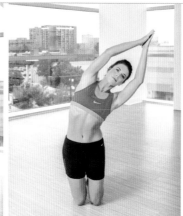

LEVEL 2

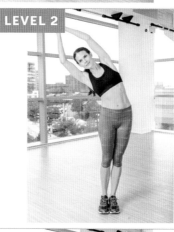

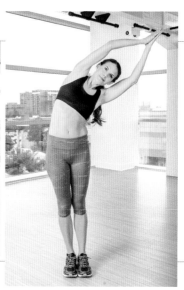

LEVEL 3

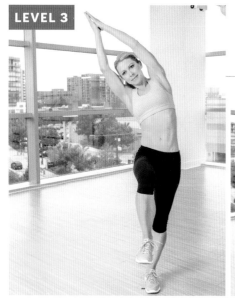

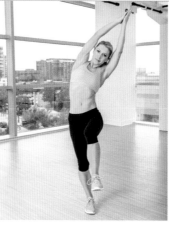

Core exercises performed from a standing position are a favorite of mine. After all, this is primarily the position from which we call upon the core muscles to work for us in daily life, and we need to train them accordingly. This particular movement also benefits your posture because it elongates the spine and helps open up the shoulders.

FROM KNEELING POSITION

▸ **1 set is 10 repetitions to each side**

Begin in a kneeling position with your knees hip-width apart. Extend your arms straight overhead and push your palms together. Shift your hips to one side while moving your hands to the opposite side, creating a "C" shape with your upper body. Go to the end of your range of motion, then come back through the center and bend in the opposite direction.

FROM STANDING POSITION

▸ **1 set is 12 repetitions to each side**

Extend your arms overhead with your palms pressed together. If you want an extra challenge, stand with your feet close together. For more stability, move your feet hip-width apart. Try not to lean forward or backward while shifting your hips into the "C" shape, alternating from side to side. Envision your body moving between two panes of glass.

FROM SINGLE LEG

▸ **1 set is 15 repetitions to each side**

Standing on one leg, extend your arms overhead and press your palms together. Shift your hips out over your stationary leg and bend to take your hands to the opposite side. Return to starting position without touching your foot down and repeat the motion to complete the set on this side, then switch sides.

TWISTING & BENDING SCULPT

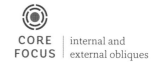

CORE FOCUS | internal and external obliques

LEVEL 1

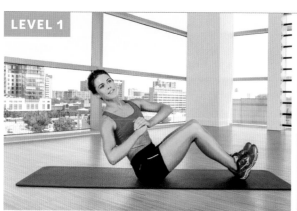
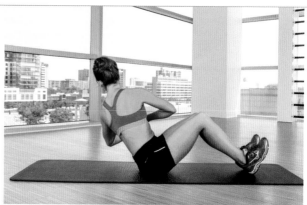

LEVEL 2

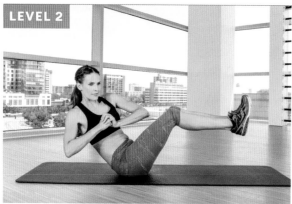
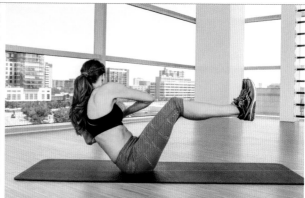

LEVEL 3

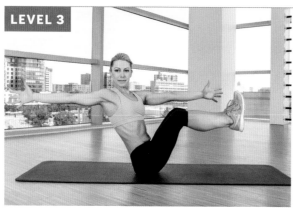
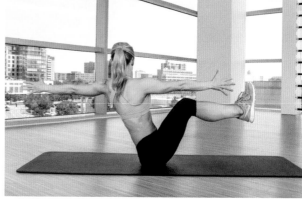

*Your core can't get enough of boat pose variations! You held the basic pose in the Balance &
Isometrics routine; then we added a leg extension to work the lower core and leg muscles in
the Pushing & Pulling routine. Now we're going to add a twisting movement to really fire up
your obliques!*

WITH HEELS ON THE GROUND   ▸ **1 set is 10 repetitions to each side**

Begin in a seated boat pose with your heels lightly touching the ground. Lift your chest and
pull your shoulder blades down and back. Make a fist with one hand, and with the opposite
hand clasp your fist and gently twist your upper body as far to one side as possible. Keep your
hands in front of your chest, twisting with your torso, not your arms. Come back through center
and twist to the opposite side. Focus on keeping your chest lifted the entire time.

WITH HEELS LIFTED   ▸ **1 set is 12 repetitions to each side**

Begin in a boat pose with your feet lifted, shins parallel to the ground. Keeping the chest
lifted, make a fist and clasp your other hand around it. Smoothly twist your torso from side
to side to reach the full extent of your range of motion. Keep your hands centered at your
chest as you work the obliques.

WITH WINDMILL ARMS   ▸ **1 set is 15 repetitions to each side**

Lean back into boat pose, lifting your shins to be parallel to the floor. Twist your torso and
extend your arms out wide, reaching toward your toes with one arm and back behind you with
the other arm. As you begin to twist to the opposite side, sweep your arms up toward the ceiling
and then down to the opposite ends of the arc. Keep your reach long and wide and your core
strong to maintain balance as you rotate your torso from side to side.

TWISTING & BENDING SCULPT

4 SIDEWINDER SERIES

LEVEL 1

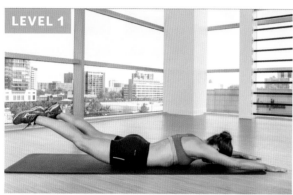
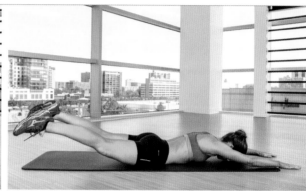

LEVEL 2

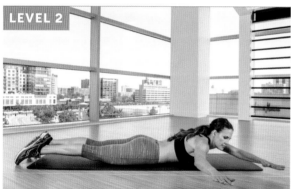
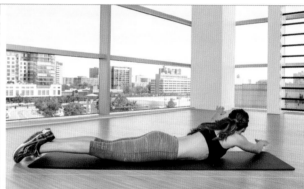

LEVEL 3

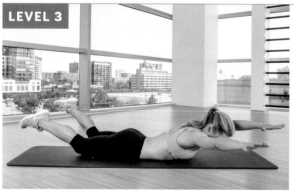
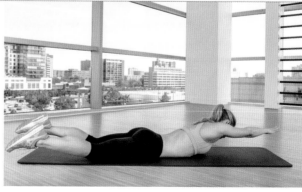

This exercise works the muscles of the back and the obliques at the same time. The movement can seem foreign the first few times you try it, but don't give up. There are many benefits to be gained from moving our bodies in a way that counters the position we spend so many hours in—slouching, with shoulders hunched forward.

MOVING LEGS

▸ **1 set is 10 repetitions to each side**

Begin by lying facedown with your arms extended overhead, pushing through your palms and forearms to anchor your upper body. Use your glutes to lift your legs and gently swing them out to one side. Move your legs back through center and out to the opposite side. This will likely begin as a smaller movement, but with practice you should be able to increase your range of motion.

MOVING ARMS

▸ **1 set is 12 repetitions to each side**

Lie facedown on the floor with your arms and legs extended. Lift your upper body off the floor about 6 inches while your legs remain anchored, pushing your quads and toes into the floor for stability. Moving only your torso and upper body, slowly sweep your arms as far as you can go to one side without moving your lower body, then sweep back through center and to the opposite side.

MOVING LEGS AND ARMS

▸ **1 set is 15 repetitions to each side**

This variation combines the upper- and lower-body movements so you can experience the sidewinding movement. Lie facedown and lift both hands and feet off the floor, pushing your weight down through your hips and torso to anchor your body. Slowly swing your hands to one side while your feet swing in the opposite direction. This will feel very unusual—you don't have to move very far in either direction to reap the benefits of this exercise. Maintaining that lift with your legs and arms, move back through center to reach the opposite sides.

TWISTING & BENDING SCULPT

SPEED SKATERS

CORE FOCUS | internal and external obliques, quadratus lumbar, spinal erectors, lateral hip muscles

LEVEL 1

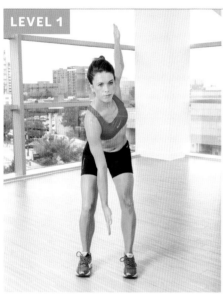

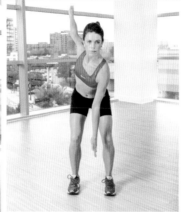

LEVEL 2

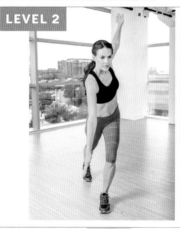

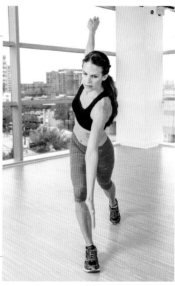

LEVEL 3

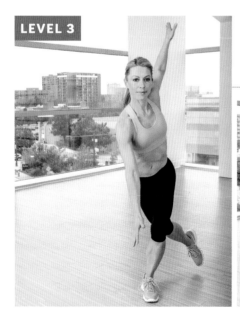

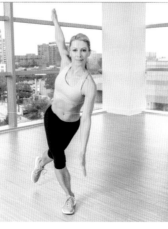

I love the speed skater movement because it calls upon the torso to twist while the lower body is working on balance and stability. This is another example of an exceptionally functional movement because it works the muscles of the core from a standing position.

STATIONARY
▸ **1 set is 10 repetitions to each side**

Begin in an athletic stance: feet hip-width apart, knees soft, arms at your sides. Lean forward at the waist and open up your arms. Twist until your arms are reaching long, from ceiling to floor. Twist only as far as you can comfortably go. Utilize the oblique muscles to do the twisting, leading from the belly button. Move back through the center and twist to the opposite side.

STEPPING FROM SIDE TO SIDE
▸ **1 set is 12 repetitions to each side**

Begin in an athletic stance: feet hip-width apart, knees soft, arms at your sides. Lean forward at the waist. Step to the side with one foot and extend the opposite foot directly behind you. As your foot reaches back to the floor behind you, open up your arms and twist until you are reaching long, from ceiling to floor. Only twist as far as your torso can comfortably go, and be sure to utilize the oblique muscles to do the twisting. Bring your back leg forward and step to the opposite side as you swing the other leg back behind your body and your arms in an arc, twisting to the other side.

JUMPING FROM SIDE TO SIDE
▸ **1 set is 15 repetitions to each side**

Speed it up! A typical speed skater movement consists of jumping from side to side, and that's exactly what you're going to do. Begin with your feet hip-width apart and knees soft, leaning forward at the waist. Instead of stepping from side to side, add a little hop and bend your knee on the landing to dip a little deeper as you open up your arms into a long twist. Repeat the motion as you jump and twist to the opposite side, settling into the rhythm of the movement. This should really get your heart rate going!

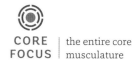

CORE FOCUS | the entire core musculature

LEVEL 1

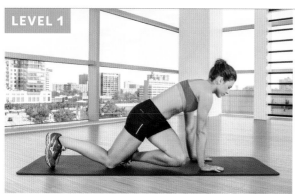
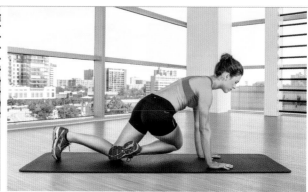

LEVEL 2

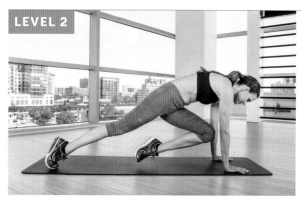
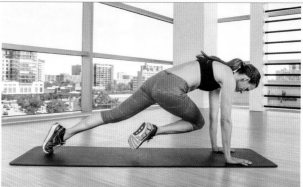

LEVEL 3

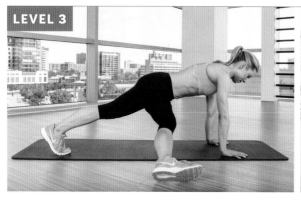
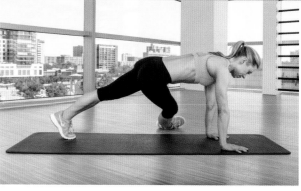

We learned the basic plank hold in the Balance & Isometrics section, and now we will use it as the foundation for movement in the lower body. I love to incorporate plank hold variations into my own routines and those of my clients because they work the front, sides, and back of the core at the same time. They also elongate the spinal column and promote good posture.

FROM KNEES
▶ **1 set is 10 repetitions to each side**

Begin in a high plank position with your knees on the floor. Keeping your belly button pulled up toward your spine and your neck long, lift one knee off the ground and sweep it under your body toward your elbow on the opposite side. Pause there before returning your knee to the starting position and repeating the movement with the opposite leg. Continue alternating legs to finish the set.

FROM TOES
▶ **1 set is 12 repetitions to each side**

By raising your knees off the floor and beginning in a high plank (or push-up) position, you challenge the muscles of your core to a greater degree. As you move your knee in toward the opposite elbow, keep the hips low and think about maintaining that extension through the back leg. Return to the starting position and repeat on the opposite side, alternating to finish the set. Remember to keep your shoulders directly over your hands throughout this exercise—a common mistake is to lean forward or backward in order to "unweight" the shoulders and make the movement easier.

WITH LEG EXTENSION
▶ **1 set is 15 repetitions to each side**

This particular variation is one of my all-time favorite core exercises. From a high plank position, reach with your leg for the opposite elbow, but this time straighten the leg out at the end of the movement and gently set it down on the floor. Repeat on the opposite side and continue alternating to finish the set. This is not only an effective core exercise but also an excellent stretch for the IT band (which runs along the outside of the thigh).

7

REVERSE TABLETOP

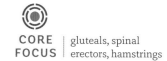

CORE FOCUS | gluteals, spinal erectors, hamstrings

LEVEL 1

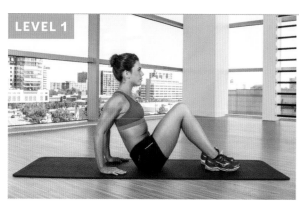

LEVEL 2

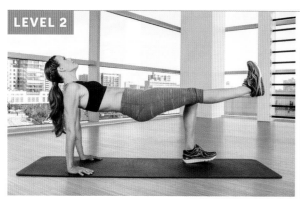

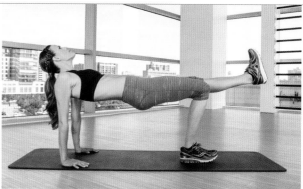

LEVEL 3

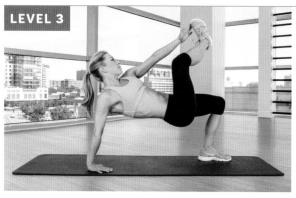

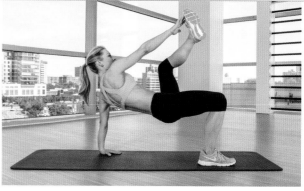

Get ready to feel the burn! The reverse tabletop is one of those movements that can feel foreign at first because the arms and legs are behind the body while the torso is pushing up toward the ceiling. Though challenging, it is an excellent way to open up the chronically tight muscles on the front side of the body while strengthening the muscles in the back.

STATIONARY

▸ **1 set is 10 repetitions**

Begin seated with your feet approximately 18–24 inches from your hips. Place your hands on the floor slightly behind you, fingertips pointing forward. Push down through your hands and feet, squeeze your glutes, and lift your hips up toward the ceiling. If you are really tight through the front of your shoulders and hips, you may find that you can't raise your hips very far. The goal is to eventually get the hips even with the knees and shoulders so that your torso forms a perfectly flat tabletop. Hold this position for a moment before lowering your hips to just above the floor, then repeat the movement until the set is complete.

WITH LEG EXTENSION

▸ **1 set is 12 repetitions on each leg**

Position your hands and feet on the floor and squeeze your glutes as you raise your hips into alignment. At the top of the movement, extend one leg out straight so it is parallel to the ground. Gently set your foot back down to the starting position and extend the opposite leg. Continue alternating legs, and try to keep your hips lifted for the full set.

WITH CROSSOVER TWIST

▸ **1 set is 15 repetitions on each leg**

Position your hands and feet on the floor and lift your hips up into a reverse tabletop position. At the top of the movement, raise one foot slowly and with control and try to reach across your body to touch your foot with the opposite hand. Return your hand and foot to the floor and repeat the movement on the opposite side. Continue alternating opposite sides to finish the set.

TWISTING & BENDING **SCULPT**

8

WINDSHIELD WIPERS

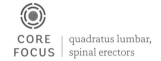

CORE FOCUS | quadratus lumbar, spinal erectors

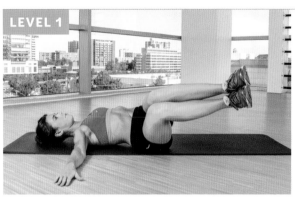

LEVEL 1

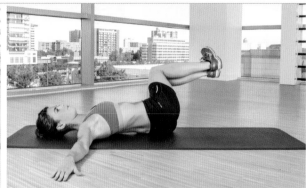

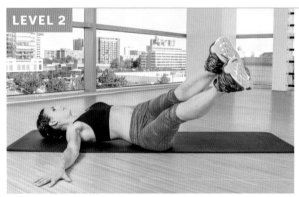

LEVEL 2

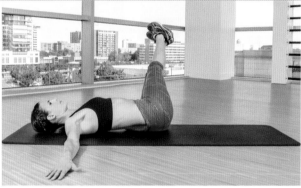

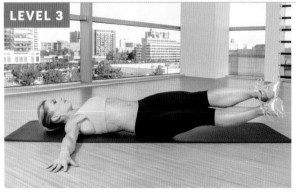

LEVEL 3

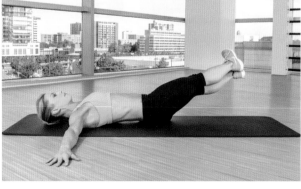

This exercise is often avoided because it works the muscles of the low back, and that can seem like dangerous territory. Your low-back muscles get stretched out and lazy thanks to chronically hunched-over posture. They need to be taxed in order to gain strength and elasticity. If you have a history of low-back injuries or pain, begin with Level 1 and don't feel compelled to drop your knees all the way to the ground. Even a few inches of side-to-side movement can begin to improve low-back strength.

WITH KNEES BENT

▸ **1 set is 10 repetitions to each side**

Begin lying down with your knees bent at a 90-degree angle, knees directly above the hips. Stretch your arms out perpendicular to your body and lower both knees to one side in a controlled movement. Using your core muscles, bring your knees back to center and then through to the opposite side.

WITH LEGS STRAIGHT

▸ **1 set is 12 repetitions to each side**

Lying on your back with your arms stretched out wide, extend both legs up straight toward the ceiling. Extend your arms out wide to anchor your body as you lower your legs to one side in a smooth movement. Go only as far as you can while still maintaining control. Lift your legs back to the upright starting position and repeat on the opposite side. If you can't get back to starting position without recruiting help from your upper body, don't drop the legs as far on the next repetition.

WITH LEGS AT 45 DEGREES

▸ **1 set is 15 repetitions to each side**

Begin by lying on your back, extending both legs up straight toward the ceiling and reaching your arms out wide to make a T. Slowly drop your legs to a point that is about 45 degrees below perpendicular. This is a longer extension and just one more way to get a twist into your torso. Lift your legs back to starting position and lower them to the opposite side.

9

PLANK WITH OBLIQUES

CORE FOCUS transverse abdominis, internal and external obliques

LEVEL 1

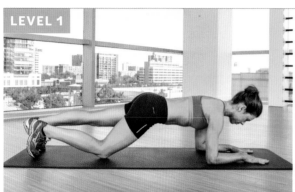

LEVEL 2

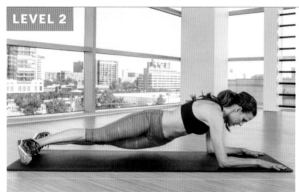

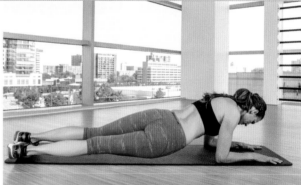

LEVEL 3

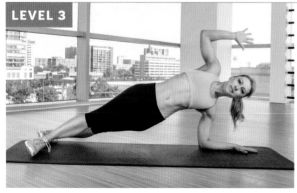

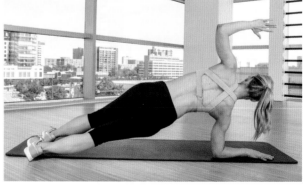

I couldn't miss the opportunity to work in one more plank exercise! This time we are getting the obliques to stretch and twist, so don't get frustrated if your hips don't make it all the way to the floor on the first few attempts. As your flexibility increases, so will your range of motion.

WITH KNEE DROPS

▸ **1 set is 10 repetitions on each side**

Begin in a basic plank hold position on your forearms with your shoulders directly over your hands, body in a straight line and low back slightly puffed out. Keeping your hips steady, gently touch one knee down to the ground. Return to starting and touch your opposite knee down. Continue alternating knees until you finish the set.

WITH HIP DROPS

▸ **1 set is 12 repetitions on each side**

Begin in basic plank position, but move your feet to be a little wider than hip width. Keeping your shoulders stable and your core engaged, pivot from your toes to the sides of your feet as you lower your hips to gently touch the floor on the same side. Come back up through center and twist to the other side, continuing in a fluid movement from side to side.

WITH ARM ROTATION

▸ **1 set is 15 repetitions on each side**

Start in basic plank position with your forearms positioned so your elbows are beneath your shoulders. Gently rotate your entire torso and lift your arm on the same side while maintaining a 90-degree angle until you are in a staggered side plank with your elbow pointing up toward the ceiling. Return back to the basic plank position and twist to the opposite side. Continue alternating sides until you finish the set.

TWISTING & BENDING   SCULPT

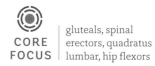

CORE
FOCUS

gluteals, spinal
erectors, quadratus
lumbar, hip flexors

LEVEL 1

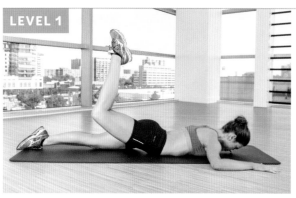

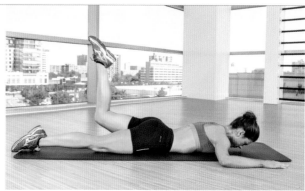

LEVEL 2

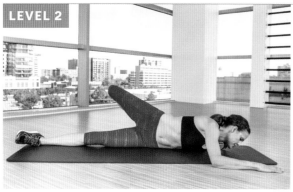

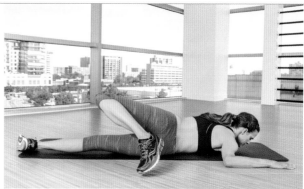

LEVEL 3

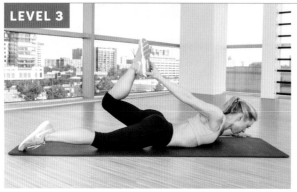

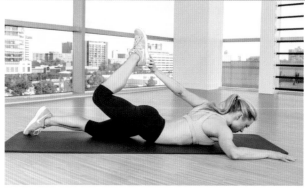

The scorpion is an exercise that I often have my clients do at the beginning of a workout to open up the front of the body while activating the glutes. Think of your body as a washcloth that you are gently wringing out.

LIFTING FOOT STRAIGHT UP ▸ 1 set is 10 repetitions on each side

Begin facedown on the floor, arms in a goalpost position. Bend one leg to form a 90-degree angle, squeeze your glute, and push that foot up toward the ceiling. Focus on engaging the glute and keeping your upper body in contact with the floor. Lower the leg to the starting position and repeat the movement with the opposite leg, alternating sides to complete the set.

WITH A TWIST ▸ 1 set is 12 repetitions on each side

This is the variation that earned this series its name. Begin facedown with your arms in a goalpost position. Lift one leg and squeeze your glute. Keeping your knee as high as possible, lift the working leg over to the opposite side of your body and try to touch the floor with your toe. Your chest will lift off the ground a little during this movement. Bring your leg back to center and repeat with the opposite leg. Continue twisting from one side to the other until you finish the set.

WITH HEEL TOUCHES ▸ 1 set is 15 repetitions on each side

Begin facedown with your arms in a goalpost position. Lift your leg, engaging the glute. Reach back with the opposite hand and try to touch your heel behind you. Return to starting position and lift the other leg, reaching back with the opposite arm. Continue alternating sides until you have finished the set.

TWISTING & BENDING SCULPT

CORE ENVY
CARDIO
Workouts

HIGH-INTENSITY INTERVAL TRAINING is the fastest, most efficient type of workout for incinerating abdominal fat. For this reason, the cardio protocol of my Core Envy program is centered around HIIT workouts. The other two types of cardio workouts you will see are Aerobic Interval Workouts and Low-Intensity Steady-State Workouts. If you do a mix of all three types of workout every week, your body will better adapt to the work you are putting in. Your cardio workouts can consist of any activity you enjoy: running, walking, biking, rowing, or dancing. Anything that gets your body working up to the designated rate of perceived exertion (RPE) is acceptable.

RULES FOR CARDIO WORKOUTS

If you have to skip a cardio day during the week, make sure it's not a HIIT workout. These should be your highest priority! Conversely, don't be tempted to make all of your cardio work high intensity. The physiological effects of overtraining are just as harmful as those of not training enough (see page 36 for details).

With all the cardio and sculpting options presented here, it might seem overwhelming to figure out how to put them together into an effective, efficient schedule. Don't worry! I've done it for you. Try to stick to the weekly schedule of cardio workouts that I have laid out in the Core Envy programs, which are outlined on pages 167–185. If you end up having to make some adjustments, use these guidelines to maintain the effectiveness of the program.

Don't eat for at least two hours before a HIIT workout. High-intensity efforts will raise your heart rate to over 70 percent of its maximum, which will decrease your rate of gastric emptying. In other words, you might end up with an upset tummy if you eat beforehand. I always do these workouts first thing in the morning on an empty stomach.

Don't do HIIT workouts on successive days. Your body needs at least 48 hours between workouts to fully recover. Pushing your heart rate into its anaerobic zone is an excellent way to burn calories and improve fitness, but it also puts stress on the body. Keep the hard workouts hard and the easy workouts easy. Working out should make your body feel empowered, not overly taxed.

Choose the level you want. I have designed the cardio programs to be completely flexible, meaning that you can perform a Level 1 workout on Monday and then step up to a Level 2 workout on Wednesday if you feel ready. Likewise, you may move down a level at any point if you feel the demands of the workout you've been following are too much. In general, the

duration and intensity of the Level 1 workouts are less than those of Level 2, which are less than those of Level 3. If you're still not sure where to start, always err on the side of choosing a lower level, knowing that you can move up whenever you choose.

Do your sculpting routine before your cardio workout. This gets your body into a fat-burning mode by the time you begin the cardio. If you're scheduled to do both on the same day, do the sculpting immediately before the cardio, if possible. If you need to break up the workouts in two time slots, then do your sculpting in the morning and your cardio later in the day (keeping in mind that your HIIT workouts should be done on a fairly empty stomach). If you absolutely must do your cardio routine first, don't worry—you'll still reap the benefits of moving your body and burning calories. Doing your core sculpting first, however, not only will burn through your readily available glycogen so that you have to rely more on fat stores during your cardio routine but also will allow you to be fresh for all of those challenging core exercises!

WORKOUT GUIDE

You will need to learn the lingo and logic of cardio workouts. Below is a quick guide to the terminology used on the following pages.

Warm-up. Increasing the core temperature of your body slowly and steadily is an important aspect of cardio workouts, especially if you're going to be working into high heart rates. Race cars are made to go from 0 to 100 mph in a very short period of time, but the human body is not. I've seen people get bored or impatient with a workout and skip the warm-up; this is dangerous because their muscles will not have enough blood rushing to them to perform the high-intensity intervals. Rev up your engine slowly so that you can perform at your best during the main set of the workout. Your warm-up doesn't have to be a different activity than your main set; it just needs to be performed at a slower pace and a lower heart rate. For example, begin with a brisk 5-minute walk or an easy jog, then move into a faster walk or run for your main set.

Main set. This is where the work starts—the portion of the workout that requires you to work the hardest and get your heart rate the highest. Below the main set intervals there are instructions that tell you whether you need to repeat the set and if there is additional rest between sets. Workouts 3 and 7 are the most complicated because they are Tabata-style workouts, and they require lots of repeats without rest. A true Tabata workout is 8 intervals of 20 seconds with a 10-second rest between each one, which is 4 minutes total. In Levels 1 and 2, you only do half of a Tabata set before you get a longer

break, but in Level 3 you get the real deal! Look for more specific instructions below these workouts to help guide you through the set.

RATE OF PERCEIVED EXERTION

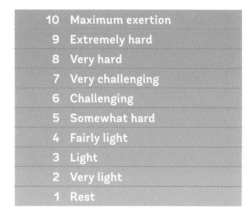

10	Maximum exertion
9	Extremely hard
8	Very hard
7	Very challenging
6	Challenging
5	Somewhat hard
4	Fairly light
3	Light
2	Very light
1	Rest

RPE. Rate of perceived exertion is measured on a scale of 1 to 10. The beauty and the potential detriment of RPE is that the number is completely subjective; you get to decide if you feel like you're working at a level 6 or a level 9. As the name implies, it is truly *perceived* exertion, and your perception might change from day to day. If you didn't sleep well or you're coming down with a cold, you might find that what felt like a 5 the day before now feels like an 8. Listen to your body and honor the feedback you're getting, but also make a commitment to being honest about how hard you're working. Most people tend to hang out between RPE 5 and 7 in almost every workout, but the real benefits of high-intensity workouts are seen in the RPE 8–9 area. Stay true to the description of RPE and make sure that your 8s are very hard and your 9s are extremely hard. You will reap great rewards from these short bursts of intensity, so make sure you aren't leaving anything on the table!

Cool-down. Very few people enjoy the cool-down portion of a workout. Much like broccoli, I know it's good for me, but I just don't like it! However, a short cool-down not only allows your body to safely return to a lower heart rate but also greatly increases the rate at which your body clears lactic acid from the bloodstream.[1] In order to reap the physiological benefits, a cool-down needs to be performed at about 35 percent of VO_2max, which equates to a 3–4 on the RPE scale.

WHAT ABOUT STRETCHING?

Entire books have been written on the topic of stretching, but here's the quick-and-dirty summary: Studies consistently show that static stretching should be performed only *after* a workout because it actually decreases muscular power, endurance, and balance. In other words, if you reach down for your toes and hold that static position for 15–30 seconds in order to stretch your hamstrings, you're actually *decreasing* the muscular power in that area.[2] This is why you should avoid static stretching before a workout.

Save your static stretches for after your workout, when it's okay for the muscles to experience decreased power and endurance. While static stretches won't necessarily help your performance during a workout, they can increase the pain tolerance in lengthening your muscles and can also result in a slightly increased range of motion.[3]

Before you happily write off stretching as the evil plot you always suspected it to be, you should know that there are different types of stretching and that not all of them carry the negative side effects of static stretching. Specifically, dynamic stretching has been shown to have positive benefits on both performance and range of motion in the muscles. Dynamic stretching is defined as movement that requires the muscles to be in constant motion and to slowly and steadily move to the endpoint of their range of motion. A slow and controlled set of walking lunges would be a good example, or gentle "toy soldier" kicks that help wake up the hamstrings. You might already be engaging in dynamic stretches throughout the day without even realizing it—if you find yourself rocking your hips from side to side or twisting your torso back and forth in your chair, that's a form of dynamic stretching.

If you have a few dynamic stretching movements that you like to do before a workout, please keep doing them. But in order to maximize your power, endurance, and balance, do static stretches only after you've completed your workout.

1
BASIC HIGH-INTENSITY INTERVALS
WORKOUT

LEVEL 1

Warm-up: 5 min. at RPE 4

Main set:
1 min. at RPE 6 / 2 min. at RPE 5
1 min. at RPE 7 / 2 min. at RPE 5
1 min. at RPE 7 / 2 min. at RPE 5
1 min. at RPE 8

Cool-down: 5 min. at RPE 4

Total time
▸ **20 min.**

Calories burned
▸ **250**

LEVEL 2

Warm-up: 5 min. at RPE 4

Main set:
1 min. at RPE 7 / 1 min. at RPE 5
1 min. at RPE 8 / 1 min. at RPE 5
1 min. at RPE 9 / 1 min. at RPE 5
Repeat set.

Cool-down: 5 min. at RPE 4

Total time
▸ **22 min.**

Calories burned
▸ **275**

LEVEL 3

Warm-up: 5 min. at RPE 4

Main set:
2 min. at RPE 7 / 1 min. at RPE 5
2 min. at RPE 8 / 1 min. at RPE 5
2 min. at RPE 9 / 1 min. at RPE 5
Repeat set.

Cool-down: 5 min. at RPE 4

Total time
▸ **28 min.**

Calories burned
▸ **325**

2 ANAEROBIC ENDURANCE INTERVALS

WORKOUT

LEVEL 1

Warm-up: 5 min. at RPE 4

Main set:
1 min. at RPE 7 / 2 min. at RPE 5
1 min. at RPE 8 / 2 min. at RPE 5
1 min. at RPE 9 / 2 min. at RPE 5
Repeat set.

Cool-down: 5 min. at RPE 4

Total time
▸ **28 min.**

Calories burned
▸ **350**

LEVEL 2

Warm-up: 5 min. at RPE 4

Main set:
1 min. at RPE 7 / 1 min. at RPE 5
1 min. at RPE 8 / 1 min. at RPE 5
1 min. at RPE 8 / 1 min. at RPE 5
1 min. at RPE 9 / 1 min. at RPE 5
1 min. at RPE 9 / 1 min. at RPE 5
Repeat set.

Cool-down: 5 min. at RPE 4

Total time
▸ **30 min.**

Calories burned
▸ **380**

LEVEL 3

Warm-up: 5 min. at RPE 4

Main set:
2 min. at RPE 7 / 1 min. at RPE 5
2 min. at RPE 8 / 1 min. at RPE 5
2 min. at RPE 8 / 1 min. at RPE 5
1 min. at RPE 9 / 1 min. at RPE 5
1 min. at RPE 9 / 1 min. at RPE 5
Repeat set.

Cool-down: 5 min. at RPE 4

Total time
▸ **36 min.**

Calories burned
▸ **420**

3 TABATA-STYLE INTERVALS

WORKOUT

LEVEL 1

Warm-up: 5 min. at RPE 4

Main set:
20 sec. at RPE 7 / 10 sec. rest
20 sec. at RPE 8 / 10 sec. rest
20 sec. at RPE 8 / 10 sec. rest
20 sec. at RPE 9 / 10 sec. rest
Rest 2 min. Repeat set.

Cool-down: 5 min. at RPE 4

Total time
▸ **18 min.**

Calories burned
▸ **225**

LEVEL 2

Warm-up: 5 min. at RPE 4

Main set:
20 sec. at RPE 7 / 10 sec. rest
20 sec. at RPE 8 / 10 sec. rest
20 sec. at RPE 9 / 10 sec. rest
20 sec. at RPE 9 / 10 sec. rest
Rest 1 min. Repeat set two
more times.

Cool-down: 5 min. at RPE 4

Total time
▸ **19 min.**

Calories burned
▸ **300**

LEVEL 3

Warm-up: 5 min. at RPE 4

Main set:
20 sec. at RPE 8 / 10 sec. rest
20 sec. at RPE 8 / 10 sec. rest
20 sec. at RPE 9 / 10 sec. rest
20 sec. at RPE 9 / 10 sec. rest
20 sec. at RPE 8 / 10 sec. rest
20 sec. at RPE 8 / 10 sec. rest
20 sec. at RPE 9 / 10 sec. rest
20 sec. at RPE 9 / 10 sec. rest
Rest 2 min. Repeat set.

Cool-down: 5 min. at RPE 4

Total time
▸ **22 min.**

Calories burned
▸ **325**

4

RECOVERY WEEK INTERVALS
WORKOUT

LEVEL 1

Warm-up: 5 min. at RPE 4

Main set:
2 min. at RPE 6 / 2 min. at RPE 5
2 min. at RPE 7 / 2 min. at RPE 5
2 min. at RPE 7

Cool-down: 5 min. at RPE 4

Total time
▸ **20 min.**

Calories burned
▸ **220**

LEVEL 2

Warm-up: 5 min. at RPE 4

Main set:
1 min. at RPE 6 / 1 min. at RPE 5
1 min. at RPE 7 / 1 min. at RPE 5
1 min. at RPE 8 / 1 min. at RPE 5
Repeat set.

Cool-down: 5 min. at RPE 4

Total time
▸ **22 min.**

Calories burned
▸ **250**

LEVEL 3

Warm-up: 5 min. at RPE 4

Main set:
2 min. at RPE 6 / 1 min. at RPE 5
2 min. at RPE 7 / 1 min. at RPE 5
2 min. at RPE 8 / 1 min. at RPE 5
Repeat set.

Cool-down: 5 min. at RPE 4

Total time
▸ **28 min.**

Calories burned
▸ **310**

5

STAIR-STEP INTERVALS

WORKOUT

LEVEL 1

Warm-up: 5 min. at RPE 4

Main set:
1 min. at RPE 6
1 min. at RPE 7
1 min. at RPE 8
2 min. at RPE 5
Repeat set 2 more times.

Cool-down: 5 min. at RPE 4

Total time
▸ **25 min.**

Calories burned
▸ **300**

LEVEL 2

Warm-up: 5 min. at RPE 4

Main set:
2 min. at RPE 7
90 sec. at RPE 8
30 sec. at RPE 9
2 min. at RPE 5
Repeat set 2 more times.

Cool-down: 5 min. at RPE 4

Total time
▸ **28 min.**

Calories burned
▸ **340**

LEVEL 3

Warm-up: 5 min. at RPE 4

Main set:
3 min. at RPE 7
2 min. at RPE 8
2 min. at RPE 9
2 min. at RPE 5
Repeat set 2 more times.

Cool-down: 5 min. at RPE 4

Total time
▸ **37 min.**

Calories burned
▸ **410**

6 | REVERSE STAIR-STEP INTERVALS
WORKOUT

LEVEL 1

Warm-up: 5 min. at RPE 4

Main set:
1 min. at RPE 6
2 min. at RPE 7
3 min. at RPE 8
2 min. at RPE 5
Repeat set.

Cool-down: 5 min. at RPE 4

Total time
‣ **26 min.**

Calories burned
‣ **290**

LEVEL 2

Warm-up: 5 min. at RPE 4

Main set:
30 sec. at RPE 7
90 sec. at RPE 8
2 min. at RPE 9
2 min. at RPE 5
Repeat set 2 more times.

Cool-down: 5 min. at RPE 4

Total time
‣ **28 min.**

Calories burned
‣ **340**

LEVEL 3

Warm-up: 5 min. at RPE 4

Main set:
1 min. at RPE 7
2 min. at RPE 8
3 min. at RPE 9
2 min. at RPE 5
Repeat set 2 more times.

Cool-down: 5 min. at RPE 4

Total time
‣ **34 min.**

Calories burned
‣ **410**

7 TURBO-CHARGED TABATA INTERVALS
WORKOUT

LEVEL 1

Warm-up: 5 min. at RPE 4

Main set:
1 min. at RPE 6 / 2 min. at RPE 5
1 min. at RPE 7 / 2 min. at RPE 5
1 min. at RPE 7 / 2 min. at RPE 5
1 min. at RPE 8

Cool-down: 5 min. at RPE 4

Total time
▸ **20 min.**

Calories burned
▸ **250**

LEVEL 2

Warm-up: 5 min. at RPE 4

Main set:
1 min. at RPE 7 / 1 min. at RPE 5
1 min. at RPE 8 / 1 min. at RPE 5
1 min. at RPE 9 / 1 min. at RPE 5
Repeat set.

Cool-down: 5 min. at RPE 4

Total time
▸ **22 min.**

Calories burned
▸ **275**

LEVEL 3

Warm-up: 5 min. at RPE 4

Main set:
2 min. at RPE 7 / 1 min. at RPE 5
2 min. at RPE 8 / 1 min. at RPE 5
2 min. at RPE 9 / 1 min. at RPE 5
Repeat set.

Cool-down: 5 min. at RPE 4

Total time
▸ **28 min.**

Calories burned
▸ **325**

1 AEROBIC BUILD INTERVALS

WORKOUT

LEVEL 1

Warm-up: 5 min. at RPE 4

Main set:
3 min. at RPE 5
3 min. at RPE 6
3 min. at RPE 7

Cool-down: 5 min. at RPE 4

Total time
▸ **19 min.**

Calories burned
▸ **200**

LEVEL 2

Warm-up: 5 min. at RPE 4

Main set:
4 min. at RPE 5
4 min. at RPE 6
4 min. at RPE 7

Cool-down: 5 min. at RPE 4

Total time
▸ **22 min.**

Calories burned
▸ **230**

LEVEL 3

Warm-up: 5 min. at RPE 4

Main set:
5 min. at RPE 5
5 min. at RPE 6
5 min. at RPE 7

Cool-down: 5 min. at RPE 4

Total time
▸ **25 min.**

Calories burned
▸ **260**

2 AEROBIC PYRAMID INTERVALS
WORKOUT

LEVEL 1

Warm-up: 5 min. at RPE 4

Main set:
3 min. at RPE 5
3 min. at RPE 6
3 min. at RPE 7
3 min. at RPE 6
3 min. at RPE 5

Cool-down: 5 min. at RPE 4

Total time
▸ **25 min.**

Calories burned
▸ **280**

LEVEL 2

Warm-up: 5 min. at RPE 4

Main set:
4 min. at RPE 5
4 min. at RPE 6
4 min. at RPE 7
4 min. at RPE 6
4 min. at RPE 5

Cool-down: 5 min. at RPE 4

Total time
▸ **30 min.**

Calories burned
▸ **330**

LEVEL 3

Warm-up: 5 min. at RPE 4

Main set:
5 min. at RPE 5
5 min. at RPE 6
5 min. at RPE 7
5 min. at RPE 6
5 min. at RPE 5

Cool-down: 5 min. at RPE 4

Total time
▸ **35 min.**

Calories burned
▸ **390**

1 LOW-INTENSITY STEADY-STATE
WORKOUT

LEVEL 1

Warm-up: 5 min. at RPE 4

Main set:
30 min. at RPE 5–6

Cool-down: 5 min. at RPE 4

Total time
▸ **40 min.**

Calories burned
▸ **400**

LEVEL 2

Warm-up: 5 min. at RPE 4

Main set:
35 min. at RPE 5–6

Cool-down: 5 min. at RPE 4

Total time
▸ **45 min.**

Calories burned
▸ **450**

LEVEL 3

Warm-up: 5 min. at RPE 4

Main set:
40 min. at RPE 5–6

Cool-down: 5 min. at RPE 4

Total time
▸ **50 min.**

Calories burned
▸ **500**

LOW-INTENSITY CARDIO

the CORE ENVY
DIET

FOR THE CORE ENVY PROGRAM TO WORK, you will need to eat fewer calories, creating a caloric deficit that leads to weight loss. When your calories are highly nutritious, you can get more out of every sculpting and cardio session and see the results in the mirror. To this end, I have created a fat-loss protocol that relies on nutritious, affordable foods that are easy to find at home or on the go—in fact, most of the Core Envy foods are readily available on restaurant menus. Of course there are countless foods that could help you achieve your goal, but by narrowing the field, I hope to make this diet less daunting and streamline the process of calorie counting. If you stick with the Core Envy foods, you can save yourself the time and trouble of hunting down nutritional information and more easily hit your daily calorie goals.

KNOW WHAT AND HOW MUCH TO EAT

To successfully execute the Core Envy Diet, you will need to know how to hit your numbers. Each day you will make sure that you eat the recommended number of servings from each food group. You will also need to know how many calories you are eating.

You are free to combine the foods in whichever way you please as long as you are meeting the daily requirements. Do that and you can then pick from your favorite foods on the list to get the rest of your calories. In my sample meal plans,

I have laid out options for three meals and two snacks each day. You'll see that there are no guidelines around when you eat these meals and snacks—at the end of the day, it comes down to calories in versus calories out. You can consume them whenever you like. That being said, most people (me included!) enjoy eating every 3–4 hours, and by eating small portions on a regular basis, you are more likely to avoid that "starving" feeling at the end of the day that often leads us to make poor dietary choices. No matter when you choose to eat, the key to a healthy, successful diet is planning. If you don't know where and how you're getting your next meal or snack, you run the risk of grabbing something convenient and unhealthy.

Calculating your DAILY CALORIC GOAL

Step 1. Calculate your resting metabolic rate by following the Mifflin equation (see page 42).

Step 2. Multiply this number by the Activity Factor to account for the level of exercise you will do on the plan (see page 42).

Step 3. Subtract 500 calories from the total to achieve weight loss.

RMR × ACTIVITY FACTOR − 500 =
YOUR DAILY CALORIC GOAL FOR WEIGHT LOSS

This is the number of calories you need to eat each day to lose 1 pound of fat every week.

Remember that no matter what number you get from the RMR equation, you should not consume fewer than 1,400 calories per day on a regular basis—your metabolism will slow down and you will run the risk of losing muscle instead of fat, which will ultimately increase your body-fat percentage. The entire purpose of the Core Envy plan is to lower your body fat and get you a sexy, lean core, so make sure you're providing your body with sufficient fuel to accomplish this goal!

CORE ENVY DAILY PORTIONS

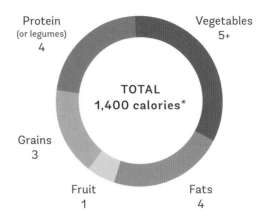

Protein (or legumes) 4

Vegetables 5+

Grains 3

Fruit 1

Fats 4

TOTAL
1,400 calories*

*Add portions as needed to hit your daily caloric goal.

For each of the foods, I have specified a portion that is equivalent to 100 calories. Thinking of your diet in 100-calorie portions makes it much easier to keep track of your calories for the day. The Core Envy Baseline template consists of 1,400 calories plus as many low-sugar veggies as you please (these are outlined on page 144). If your goal is 1,700 calories, then you would start by eating the portions noted in the baseline template and add three more portions from the Core Envy foods list to get the extra 300 calories. Pretty easy, right?

Vegetables are the primary focus of the Core Envy nutrition plan. Highly nutritious yet low in calories, vegetables add up to weight loss. Almost all the veggies included in my list are so low in calories and sugar that you can eat unlimited amounts of

them and not have to worry about counting those calories. Vegetables that are naturally higher in calories—such as Brussels sprouts, carrots, and peas—while still nutritious, must be counted toward your daily caloric intake. If you want to avoid fretting over servings with your veggies, simply focus on those listed as "zero calories" in the chart. Your goal is a minimum of 5 servings of vegetables every day. By simply eating a vegetable with every meal and snack, this goal should be easy. Make vegetables a priority when choosing what to eat. Pick your veggies first, then fill in the rest of your plate around them. Once you have your vegetables, the rest of your calories will come from a nice balance of fruit, lean protein, healthy fats, and whole-grain carbohydrates.

CORE ENVY FOODS

FOOD	100-CALORIE PORTION
LOW-SUGAR VEGETABLES	
Asparagus	▸ Unlimited - count as zero calories
Broccoli	▸ Unlimited
Cabbage	▸ Unlimited
Cauliflower	▸ Unlimited
Leafy greens: kale, spinach, arugula, collard greens, chard, etc.	▸ Unlimited
Peppers: red, yellow, orange	▸ Unlimited
Tomatoes, fresh	▸ Unlimited
HIGHER-CALORIE VEGETABLES	
Brussels sprouts	▸ 10 sprouts
Carrots	▸ 4 small, 6" long
Peas	▸ 1 cup
FRUITS	
Apples	▸ 1 medium, 3" diameter
Bananas	▸ 1 small, 6" long
Blueberries	▸ 1 cup
Grapefruit	▸ 1 medium, 3" diameter
Oranges	▸ 1 large, 3" diameter
Strawberries	▸ 2 cups (whole, uncut)
PROTEIN	
Beef: organic, grass-fed, at least 90% lean	▸ 2 oz.
Chicken breast: organic, free-range	▸ 3 oz. cooked
Eggs: organic, free-range	▸ 1½ whole eggs or 5 egg whites
Seafood: cod, salmon, tuna, halibut, tilapia	▸ 2 oz. cooked salmon or 3 oz. cooked white fish
Shellfish: clams, oysters, crab	▸ 4 oz. cooked
Turkey breast: organic, no added nitrates	▸ 3 oz. cooked

FOOD	100-CALORIE PORTION
FATS	
Almonds	▸ ½ oz., about 12 almonds
Avocado	▸ ⅓ avocado
Olive oil	▸ Slightly less than 1 Tbsp.
Peanuts	▸ ½ oz., about 17 peanuts
Pistachios	▸ 1 oz. shelled or ½ cup unshelled
Sunflower seeds	▸ ½ oz. shelled or ⅓ cup unshelled
GRAINS & CARBOHYDRATES	
Brown rice	▸ ⅛ cup uncooked or ½ cup cooked
Oats	▸ ¼ cup uncooked
Polenta	▸ 3½-inch slices or ½ cup uncooked
Quinoa	▸ ⅛ cup uncooked or ¾ cup cooked
Squash: acorn, butternut, spaghetti	▸ 1½ cups cubed (acorn, butternut) or 2½ cups cooked (spaghetti)
Sweet potatoes/Yams	▸ ⅔ cup cooked
LEGUMES	
Black beans	▸ ½ cup cooked
Chickpeas	▸ ⅓ cup cooked
Lentils	▸ ½ cup cooked
Pinto beans	▸ ½ cup cooked
Tofu	▸ 6 oz. soft or 5 oz. firm

If you want to simplify the calorie counting, follow the sample meal plans that I have put together for you. These plans assume a total of 1,400 calories a day, so if your personal number is higher than that, you will need to add the appropriate number of portions. In the guidelines for how to utilize the meal plans, I've included some helpful hints for how to choose which foods to add. I have made every effort to keep the meals straightforward and easy to prepare; in several instances there is an "on-the-go" option that lets you stay on the plan when you're running out the door or don't feel like cooking. On the flip side, if you love trying new recipes, I encourage you to follow some of the slimming recipes that I've created. You can make enough to feed your whole family or use the leftovers to get more out of your time spent in the kitchen These meals are so delicious that you will find it hard to believe they are so good for you!

DRINK PLENTY OF WATER!

To have a lean body, you need to eat healthy foods in the right quantities, but you also need to be well-hydrated. I learned firsthand about the importance of hydration in my own pursuit of an enviable core. One of my first mentors in the personal training field competed in bodybuilding competitions. He was an expert at manipulating body composition, and I watched him coach his clients through dietary changes that produced astounding results. One of his most important rules for fat loss was hydration. At the time I thought this seemed counterintuitive—wouldn't I feel bloated and bogged down with water weight if I drastically increased my water intake? As it turns out, not drinking enough water can actually cause your body to store more fat, and here's why:[1]

- ▶ The body can mistake thirst for hunger, meaning that it will signal you to eat when you really need to drink water.
- ▶ Chronic dehydration causes your metabolism to slow down in order to conserve water and energy, which also causes your liver to store more fat.
- ▶ Dehydration places stress on the body, signaling it to release insulin and cortisol, both of which cause the body to store extra fat.

In order to ensure adequate hydration, you should aim for a number of ounces that is half the number of pounds of your body weight each day (for example, if you weigh 150 pounds, you should drink 75 ounces per day). If you sweat a lot during your workouts, you will need to drink even more to replace that loss in water. A general rule is to add 20 ounces for each hour of intense workout.

KEEP A
FOOD JOURNAL

A few years back, I worked with a woman in her late 40s who came to me in desperation. She was consistently eating clean, healthy foods, yet she could not lose the 15 pounds she had put on since having her two children 10 years earlier. I asked her to keep a food journal so that I could figure out which items were the culprits. Week after week, she submitted one of the healthiest, most calorie-conscious food journals I have ever seen. She was working out regularly, including three days a week of fat-incinerating interval routines, yet the pounds wouldn't budge. We removed dairy from her diet, and the pounds stayed on. We eliminated corn and soy products, added water, added fiber, and drastically cut sodium, but the scale didn't move a tenth of a pound. I was frustrated that I couldn't figure it out, and my client was frustrated that she was working harder and harder and still not seeing results. Eventually she decided to stop training with me. I felt defeated.

Several years later I ran into her at the grocery store. It was obvious that she had finally dropped the weight—she looked lean and healthy. I had to know how she had done it. She looked me in the eye and said, "I quit lying in my food journal."

Be honest about what and how much you're eating. If you grab a few M&Ms from your colleague's candy bowl, write it down.

YOUR METRICS FOR WEIGHT LOSS

- ▶ Stay within your daily calorie goal by tracking your food.

- ▶ Eat at least one portion of vegetables with each meal/snack.

- ▶ Drink half your body weight in ounces every day.

If you munch on some chips while you're preparing dinner, write it down. Your weight-loss efforts will pay off if you avoid mindless eating and a few extra bites here and there.

To help guide you in keeping track of your daily calories, I've created a Core Envy log (page 190) that makes it easy to check off the baseline requirements and fill in the rest of the day's calories. Review the sample that follows and use the method that works best for you. At the end of every week, check your measurements. There's a chart for tracking your body composition and waist, hip, and belly-button measurements (page 188). It might take a few weeks for your waistline to begin to tell the story of how hard you've been working. Be warned that if you lie in your food journal, your weekly measurements will deliver the hard truth.

HOW TO CHEAT
AND WIN

You might be wondering if there's room for the occasional indulgence—a small piece of chocolate, a glass of wine, anything at all?

CORE ENVY LOG

Date 6/7   Water (8 oz.) 1̶ 2̶ 3̶ 4̶ 5̶ 6̶ 7̶ 8̶

DIET

Breakfast — Core Envy Smoothie

Snack — 2 hard-boiled eggs with
    1 cup broccoli

Lunch — Chicken Salad from Chipotle with
    corn, 3/4 cup brown rice

Snack — Kind Bar (count as 1 fat, 1 grain)

Dinner — Baked Halibut with Strawberry
    Cilantro Salad and 3/4 cup brown rice

FOOD	PORTION	CALORIES
Vegetables	1̶ 2̶ 3̶ 4̶ 5̶ 6 7	200
Fruits	1̶ 2̶ 3	150 (1½ fruit)
Protein (including legumes)	1̶ 2̶ 3̶ 4̶ 5 6 7	400
Fats	1̶ 2̶ 3̶ 4 5	300
Grains & Carbohydrates	1̶ 2̶ 3̶ 4̶	400

	DAILY CALORIE GOAL	1500
	ACTUAL CALORIES	1450
	+1⊝	50

WORKOUT

SCULPTING

ROUTINE	SETS	EXERCISES	LEVEL
Pushing + Pulling	2	1–10	2

CARDIO

WORKOUT	NO.	TIME	LEVEL
Aerobic Intervals	1	22 min.	2

In fact, I encourage you to enjoy "cheating" once a week. I don't believe in following a diet protocol that is so rigid that there is literally no room for error; this is dangerous both physically and mentally. You need to have a plan that is sustainable on a daily basis and that you can adhere to for the long term, not just a crash weight-loss program that is too extreme to follow for more than a few days. For these reasons, I want you to have the luxury of looking forward to a little indulgence once a week, knowing that you have worked hard to earn it.

There's just one caveat—if you overdo it on your cheat meal, you could ruin all the progress you made in the previous six days. If this sounds overly dramatic or calorically impossible, think about the cheat meals that you have enjoyed in the past. Based on both my own failed diet attempts and those of my clients, it could look something like this:

▶ Basket of warm bread with butter or olive oil on every slice (500–700 calories)
▶ 3 pieces of sausage-and-mushroom pizza with thick crust (800–1,000 calories)
▶ 3 glasses of red wine, 6 ounces each (450 calories)
▶ Large piece of cheesecake with whipped cream (1,000–1,200 calories)

If you were to eat all of this in one sitting, it would add up to as much as 3,350 calories! If a daily 500-calorie deficit is the goal, that amounts to a 3,500-calorie deficit each week. Our hypothetical cheat meal is dangerously close to 3,500 calories, effectively zeroing out the caloric restriction that you worked so hard to create.

I've seen cheat meals sabotage progress more times than I can count. To avoid this scenario, cash in your weekly cheat for a single food, not an entire meal. This means your cheat will consist of a couple hundred calories rather than a couple thousand. Stay focused on obtaining an enviable core, and don't let the concept of a cheat meal equate to a carte blanche for consumption.

READY-MADE MEAL PLANS

These plans are based on a 1,400-calorie diet, so if your personal caloric intake that you calculated using the formula on page 142 is higher, then you'll need to add the appropriate number of 100-calorie portions to reach your final goal. You might find yourself wondering which types of foods to choose to get to your number. Here are a few basic guidelines to help you decide:

▶ If you're following the Level 3 cardio plans and are generally very active, add a combination of carbohydrates and fats.
▶ If you want a little treat after dinner or are craving something sweet, add fruit.
▶ If you want to stabilize your blood sugar or work on lean muscle and toning, add protein or legumes.

HOW TO USE THE MEAL PLANS

▶ **Each breakfast, lunch & dinner** option equals approximately **300 calories.** Each snack option equals approximately 200.

▶ **Choose 1 breakfast, 1 lunch, 1 dinner & 2 snacks each day.** This will total 1,300–1,400 calories. If your personal daily caloric intake is higher, add another snack or another meal to get to your number.

▶ **If you want to eat the same breakfast every day, go for it!** Consistency is key, especially when you're first starting the Core Envy program.

▶ **When possible, make your lunch** from dinner leftovers the night before. Cook once and eat twice . . . or maybe three or four times!

▶ **Each recipe lists the number of total calories** as well as the number of Core Envy food portions, allowing you to easily keep track of how many veggies, fruits, proteins, fats, grains, and legumes you're getting each day.

▶ **Don't forget to enjoy a cheat item one or two times a week!** Your cheat food should be no more than 400 calories maximum. The rest of your day needs to follow the Core Envy Diet protocol.

BREAKFAST	SNACKS	LUNCH	DINNER
OPTION 1 Core Envy Smoothie (page 153)	**OPTION 1** ⅓ cup Sweet and Spicy Hummus and unlimited zero- calorie veggies (page 164)	**OPTION 1** Tofu Spring Rolls with Peanut Sauce (page 157)	**OPTION 1** Baked Halibut with Strawberry Cilantro Salsa (page 162)
OPTION 2 Veggie Omelet (page 152)	**OPTION 2** 2 hard-boiled eggs and unlimited zero-calorie veggies	**OPTION 2** Core Envy Power Salad (page 156)	**OPTION 2** Baked Chicken Breast with Butternut Squash with side of brown rice (page 160)
OPTION 3 Sweet Potato Scramble (page 154)	**OPTION 3** 2 Tbsp. nuts and unlimited zero- calorie veggies	**OPTION 3** Bunless Turkey Burger with Large Salad (page 158)	**OPTION 3** Broccoli Quinoa with Beef Tenderloin Tips (page 161)
OPTION 4 Mini-Quiches with side of fruit (page 155)	**OPTION 4** Kind Bar or any other bar less than 200 calories and 5 grams sugar	**OPTION 4** Sweet Potato and Black Bean Taco Bowl (page 159)	**OPTION 4** Salmon with Polenta Cakes and Green Beans (page 163)
ON-THE-GO OPTION 1 hard-boiled egg, 1 Green Machine drink by Naked (no-sugar-added variety)	(All snack options qualify as on-the- go options because they are easy to transport.)	**ON-THE-GO OPTION** Chicken salad from Chipotle (lettuce, chicken, mild salsa, half portion of corn, no dressing)	**ON-THE-GO OPTION** 1 sushi roll (approx. 6 pieces) with tuna or salmon, avocado, cucumber (no cream cheese, no fried rolls), side salad with 2 Tbsp. vinaigrette dressing

MEAL PLANS DIET

VEGGIE OMELET *Makes 1 serving*

Omelets made with egg whites will save you calories and fat. I purchase egg whites in a separate carton because the convenience is worth the cost for me, especially since I eat egg whites almost every day!

1½ tsp. olive oil or olive oil cooking spray

1 whole egg plus 2 egg whites, lightly beaten

1 cup fresh spinach, chopped

¼ cup mushrooms, sliced

Any other vegetables of your choice

1 tsp. Italian seasoning

1 portion of fruit on the side

1 Bring a skillet to medium heat as you lightly coat the bottom of the pan with olive oil. Add the eggs, tipping the pan to spread them evenly. Cook for 2 minutes, gently lifting the edges of the egg as it firms up.

2 Add the spinach, mushrooms, and Italian seasoning and cook for another 2 to 3 minutes or until eggs are completely cooked. Fold the omelet in half and serve alongside fresh fruit.

Per serving ▶ 270 calories (includes 1 apple on the side)

Portions ▶ 1 vegetable, 1 fruit, 1½ protein, ½ fat

CORE ENVY SMOOTHIE *Makes 2 servings*

This smoothie may be green in color, but the banana overwhelms any bitterness that may arise from the veggies. Feel free to add any other veggies you may have in your fridge: tomatoes, peppers, broccoli, etc. Be creative and find your favorite flavor!

2 cups raw spinach or other leafy greens

1 cup broccoli

1 cup blueberries

2 scoops vanilla protein powder
(I recommend Vega brand)

1 Tbsp. peanut butter

1 medium banana

2 cups ice water

1 Throw all the ingredients in a blender or food processor and hit puree.

TIP: You can store the leftover smoothie in a covered mason jar in the fridge—it makes for an easy snack later in the day or postworkout.

Per serving ▸ 300 calories

Portions ▸ 1 vegetable, 1 fruit, 1 protein, 1 fat

SWEET POTATO
SCRAMBLE *Makes 2 servings*

1¹/₂ Tbsp. olive oil

1 clove garlic, minced

2 Tbsp. onion, diced

1 medium sweet potato, cubed

2 cups fresh spinach, chopped

2 whole eggs, plus 2 whites

¹/₄ tsp. paprika (optional)

Pinch of cayenne pepper (optional)

1 Bring a skillet to medium heat. Add the olive oil, garlic, onion, and sweet potato. Stir consistently to keep the garlic and onion from burning.

2 When sweet potatoes begin to soften, add the spinach and egg as well as paprika and cayenne if you like. Continue to stir until eggs are cooked through. Add salt and pepper to taste.

Per serving ▸ 290 calories

Portions ▸ 1 vegetable, 1 protein, 1 grain, 1 fat

MINI-QUICHES *Makes 4 servings*

2 Tbsp. olive oil

6 whole eggs

5 egg whites

2½ oz. goat cheese

1 cup spinach, chopped

1 cup tomatoes, diced

½ cup mushrooms, sliced

Salt, pepper, fresh or dried basil

---

1 Preheat oven to 350 degrees. Drizzle the olive oil evenly over the bottom of 12 muffin tins.

2 Mix together whole eggs, egg whites, and goat cheese, whisking gently. Add the spinach, tomatoes, and mushrooms to the bottom of the tins, then pour the egg mixture on top. Leave about 1 inch of space at the top of each tin. Sprinkle salt, pepper, and basil on top of each egg mixture.

3 Bake for 25 minutes or until the centers of the mini-quiches are cooked through. Serve with 1 portion of fruit.

TIP: These quiches keep well in the refrigerator or freezer. Once thawed, just heat for 60 seconds in the microwave before serving.

Per serving ▸ 300 calories (3 quiches plus 1 portion fruit)

Portions ▸ 1 vegetable, 1 fruit, 1½ protein, 1 fat

CORE ENVY
POWER SALAD *Makes 2 servings*

1¹/₂ tsp. olive oil

8 oz. skinless chicken breast
(raw measurement)

Salt and pepper to taste

4 cups mixed greens

1 Granny Smith apple, unpeeled and
cut into small chunks

2 oz. goat cheese

2 Tbsp. walnuts, finely chopped

1 lemon, juiced

---

1 Season the chicken breast with salt and
pepper and cook on medium heat on the
grill for approximately 8 minutes each side,
or until the center is no longer pink.

2 Meanwhile, assemble the rest of the
salad ingredients in a large bowl.

3 Remove the chicken breast from the
grill when it's finished cooking, cut into
1-inch chunks, and add to the top of the
salad. Top with a squeeze of fresh lemon
juice and a little salt and pepper to taste.

Per serving ▸ 318 calories

Portions ▸ 1 vegetable, ¹/₂ fruit, 2 protein, 1 fat

TOFU **SPRING ROLLS**
WITH PEANUT SAUCE *Makes 2 servings*

I love these spring rolls because they take seconds to make, they refrigerate well, and they're a perfect snack food that's healthy and filling. Double the recipe if you want to have leftovers.

1½ cups cooked brown rice

4 round brown-rice papers

4 oz. extra-firm organic tofu, sliced into French-fry-like strips

1 cup chopped spinach, mixed greens, or combination

¼ cup grated carrot

¼ cup chopped fresh cilantro

2 Tbsp. gluten-free peanut sauce for dipping (I recommend San-J brand)

1   Cook the brown rice according to the instructions on the package (you can make as much rice as you want and use the leftovers for another day).

2   Dunk each individual rice paper in a pie pan filled with warm water for 10–15 seconds. This will make the rice paper soft and pliable.

3   Lay the softened rice paper on a clean work surface. Place 1 slice tofu, ¼ cup spinach, and 1 tablespoon of carrot and cilantro in the center of the paper. Roll the rice paper up like a burrito. Wet your fingertips to create a seal. Place the finished spring roll seam-side-down as you repeat this process with the remaining rice paper.

4   Cover the completed spring rolls with plastic wrap, then refrigerate for 30 minutes to chill the rice paper. Serve with a side of gluten-free peanut sauce for dipping and ¾ cup cooked brown rice.

Per serving ▸ 306 calories (2 rolls, 1 Tbsp. peanut sauce, ¾ cup cooked rice)

Portions ▸ 1 vegetable, 1 protein, 1 grain, 1 fat

BUNLESS TURKEY BURGER
WITH LARGE SALAD *Makes 4 servings*

FOR THE TURKEY BURGER:

1 lb. extra-lean ground turkey breast

2 cloves minced garlic

1 Tbsp. gluten-free soy sauce

1/2 tsp. ground pepper

1/4 tsp. cayenne (optional)

4 slices fresh tomato (optional)

4 whole leaves fresh basil (optional)

---

1 Combine turkey, garlic, soy sauce, pepper, and cayenne in a large glass bowl. Knead with your hands until all ingredients are combined. Divide into four equal portions and form into patties.

2 Cook the burgers on medium-high heat on a grill for 6–7 minutes each side or until centers are no longer pink. Serve with a slice of fresh tomato and basil and your choice of salsa, mustard, or sugar-free ketchup.

FOR THE SALAD:

Any combination of leafy green veggies from the Core Envy foods list

16 small cherry tomatoes

2 cups blueberries

2 Tbsp. balsamic vinegar

2 Tbsp. fresh lemon juice

1/4 cup olive oil

---

1 Combine the leafy greens, cherry tomatoes, and blueberries in a bowl.

2 Whisk together the remaining ingredients for the dressing; pour over the salad mixture and toss until evenly distributed.

Per serving ▸ 290 calories

Portions ▸ 2 vegetable, 1/2 fruit, 1 1/2 protein, 1 fat

SWEET POTATO AND BLACK BEAN
TACO BOWL _Makes 4 servings_

1½ tsp. olive oil

2 cloves garlic, finely chopped

¼ cup onions, chopped

1 large sweet potato, chunked

1 cup red pepper, chopped

1 15-oz. can black beans, drained

1 packet all-natural taco seasoning (no MSG)

4 cups shredded lettuce

1 avocado, sliced

Ready-made salsa, no added sugar (optional)

Fresh cilantro (optional)

1 Heat olive oil in a large skillet over medium-high heat. Add garlic and onions and stir for a few minutes until golden in color. Add the sweet potato and red pepper and continue to cook until both start to soften.

2 Reduce the heat to low and add taco seasoning as specified on the packaging. Then add the black beans, stirring until the mixture is heated through and taco seasoning has been fully incorporated.

3 To serve, place 1 cup of shredded lettuce in a large bowl. Top with one-quarter of the sweet potato mixture and sliced avocado, then add salsa and cilantro if you like.

Per serving ▶ 320 calories

Portions ▶ 1 grain, 1 legume, 1 fat

BAKED CHICKEN BREAST
WITH BUTTERNUT SQUASH *Makes 8 servings*

4 cups butternut squash, peeled and cut into 1-inch cubes

2 medium Granny Smith apples, peeled and coarsely chopped

3/4 cup white onion, chopped

1/2 cup walnuts, finely chopped

2 Tbsp. olive oil

1 tsp. cinnamon

1/2 tsp. sea salt

1/4 tsp. black pepper

2 lb. boneless, skinless chicken breast

1 Preheat oven to 350 degrees.

2 Combine everything except the chicken in a 9 × 13–inch baking dish and toss until well blended.

3 Place the chicken breast in a separate baking dish and season with salt, pepper, garlic, and any other sugar-free seasoning you prefer.

4 Place the squash dish in the oven to bake for 25 minutes. Stir the squash dish and return it to the oven along with the chicken dish. Continue to bake both dishes for 25–30 minutes or until chicken is no longer pink in the center.

5 Slice the cooked chicken into 8 equal portions and serve alongside 1 cup of the roasted squash, apple, and walnut mixture.

Per serving ▸ 320 calories

Portions ▸ 1 vegetable, 1/4 fruit, 2 protein, 1/4 grain, 1 fat

BROCCOLI QUINOA WITH
BEEF TENDERLOIN TIPS *Makes 6 servings*

1 cup quinoa, uncooked

5 cups broccoli florets and stems, cut small

2 cloves garlic

2/3 cup sliced almonds

1/8 tsp. sea salt

2 Tbsp. fresh lemon juice

3 Tbsp. olive oil

1/4 cup low-fat coconut milk

1 lb. beef tenderloin steak

1 Cook the quinoa according to the instructions on the packaging and set it aside.

2 Bring a small amount of water to a simmer in a large pot, then add the salt and broccoli florets and stems. Cover and cook for 1 minute. Immediately remove from heat, strain, and run under cold water so the broccoli stops cooking.

3 In a food processor or blender, combine 2 cups of the cooked broccoli, garlic, 1/2 cup almonds, salt, and lemon juice. Begin to pulse this mixture, adding the olive oil and coconut milk between pulses. Continue pulsing until the mixture is smooth like a pesto.

4 Combine the quinoa with 1/2 cup of the pesto you just made. Add the remaining broccoli florets. Adjust the flavor by adding more broccoli pesto if you like and seasoning with salt and pepper.

5 To prepare the beef tenderloin, first trim any fat. Season with salt and pepper and set aside. Lightly coat a large skillet with olive oil cooking spray. Over medium heat, cook the steak for 7–8 minutes on each side. Remove from heat and let rest for 5 minutes before cutting into 6 equal portions.

6 To serve, place 3/4 cup broccoli quinoa on each plate and sprinkle with the remaining almonds. Serve with a slice of the beef tenderloin.

Per serving ▶ 350 calories (3/4 cup broccoli quinoa plus 2 oz. beef)

Portions ▶ 1 vegetable, 1 grain, 2 fat, 1 protein

BAKED HALIBUT WITH STRAWBERRY CILANTRO SALSA *Makes 4 servings*

1 Tbsp. olive oil

1 Tbsp. fresh lemon juice

1 tsp. sea salt

1 tsp. black pepper

1 lb. fresh halibut steaks
(cut into 4 pieces)

1½ cups brown rice

2 tomatoes, chopped

Juice from half a lime

½ avocado, diced

½ red onion, diced

6 strawberries, chopped

1 Tbsp. cilantro, finely chopped

½ tsp. cayenne pepper

½ Tbsp. olive oil

---

1 Combine the olive oil, lemon juice, salt, and pepper and pour over the halibut in a glass dish. Cover and allow to marinate in the refrigerator for at least 30 minutes.

2 Cook the brown rice according to the instructions on the package.

3 Preheat the oven to 450 degrees.

4 Remove the fish from the refrigerator and set on the counter for 10 minutes to allow the glass dish to come to room temperature. After 10 minutes, place the glass dish (with the marinade still on the fish) in the oven. Bake for 8–12 minutes, depending on the thickness of the fish. Remove when fish flakes easily with a fork.

5 While the fish is in the oven, combine the remaining ingredients in a large bowl to create the salsa.

6 Serve each piece of fish over ¾ cup cooked brown rice with salsa divided into 4 equal amounts.

Per serving ▸ 330 calories (¾ cup cooked rice, 1 piece fish, salsa)

Portions ▸ ½ fruit, 1 protein, 1 grain, 1 fat

SALMON WITH POLENTA CAKES AND GREEN BEANS Makes 4 servings

12 oz. wild-caught salmon

1 Tbsp. fresh lemon juice

1/4 tsp. cayenne pepper (optional)

Salt and pepper

FOR THE POLENTA CAKES:

1 Tbsp. olive oil

1 18-oz. tube of premade polenta, cut into 1/2-inch slices

1/4 tsp. dried oregano

1/4 tsp. dried basil

Salt and pepper

Fresh green beans

---

1 Preheat the broiler to high.

2 Place the salmon on a baking sheet lined with foil and drizzle with lemon juice. Season with cayenne pepper, salt, and pepper to your liking. Broil the salmon for 10–12 minutes or until the center is no longer brightly colored. Do not flip or turn the salmon while broiling.

3 While the salmon is cooking, prepare the polenta and green beans.

4 Heat olive oil in a large skillet over medium heat. Gently place the polenta slices in the skillet and sprinkle the spices on top. Allow each slice to cook until deeply golden brown on each side.

5 For the green beans, place as many fresh green beans as you like in a steamer pot and steam for approximately 10–15 minutes or until they reach desired tenderness.

6 Divide the salmon, polenta, and green beans into 4 equal servings and enjoy!

Per serving ▸ 340 calories

Portions ▸ 1 vegetable, 1 1/2 protein, 1 grain, 1 fat

SWEET AND SPICY
HUMMUS *Makes 9 servings*

This variation on a traditional hummus has a bit of a kick. If you prefer your hummus with a more neutral taste, simply leave out the cayenne pepper. Adjust the ingredients to suit your taste. For example, you may like more garlic and less tahini or more cayenne (spicy!) and less cinnamon. Have fun and be creative!

1 15-oz. can chickpeas

$1/3$ cup tahini

2 Tbsp. fresh lemon juice

2 Tbsp. olive oil

$1/8$ tsp. black pepper

$1/8$ tsp. sea salt

$1/8$ tsp. cinnamon

$1/4$ tsp. cayenne pepper

2 cloves minced garlic

1 Reserve $1/2$ cup liquid from the chickpeas, then drain and rinse.

2 Put all ingredients (including the reserved liquid from the chickpeas) in a blender or food processor and blend until a creamy texture is reached.

Per serving ▶ 114 calories ($1/3$ cup)

Portions ▶ $1/2$ fat, $1/2$ legume

the Core Envy
WORKOUT PLAN

the 8-week
WORKOUT PLAN

NOW IT'S TIME to put all of the sculpting routines and cardio workouts into a weekly schedule. Don't worry; you won't have to figure out how to best design a workout program—I've done it all for you! In the following pages you will find an 8-week guide to the Core Envy program.

The progression of intensity in these weekly schedules is based on researched principles of exercise science, and I strongly encourage you to stick to the parameters even if you're tempted to throw something together on your own. I have carefully alternated high-intensity and low-intensity days and have strategically placed rest days when your body will need them most. In addition, there is a science to the 8-week progression: Weeks 1–3 will see a gradual increase in intensity and duration, then Week 4 will allow you to recover from your hard work, and then the cycle is repeated again. In this manner you will build core strength and endurance without overtaxing your body.

There are three program levels to choose from: Level 1 is moderate, Level 2 is intermediate, and Level 3 is advanced. If you're not sure which one is best for you, I suggest erring on the easier side; you can always bump up to the next level after your first few workouts if you feel they're not challenging enough. I also realize that people are often not at the same level for both cardio and sculpting, which can result in someone being at a Level 3 for cardio workouts but a Level 1 for core strength (or vice versa). *If your core strength and cardio strength are not at the same level, follow the weekly program that is in line with your core strength.*

I have arranged the cardio workouts so that each day designates which cardio routine to follow (i.e., HIIT Workout 1), but it does not specify which workout level to follow. This means you can follow the Level 1 program for core strength, but you can choose the Level 3 cardio workout. Additional instructions and explanations accompany each week's schedule.

RULES FOR WORKOUTS

▶ **If you have to skip a cardio day during the week, make sure it's not a HIIT workout.** These should be your highest priority! Conversely, don't be tempted to make all of your cardio work high intensity. **The physiological effects of overtraining are just as harmful as those of not training enough.**

▶ **Don't do HIIT workouts on successive days.** Your body needs at least 48 hours between workouts to fully recover.

▶ **Choose the level you want.** I have designed the **cardio programs to be completely flexible,** meaning that you can perform a Level 1 workout on Monday and then step up to a Level 2 workout on Wednesday if you feel ready. **Within the sculpting routines, choose the appropriate level** for each exercise.

▶ **Do your sculpting routine before your cardio workout.** This gets your body into a **fat-burning** mode by the time you begin the cardio.

▶ **When doing sculpting exercises,** don't rush the movement. **Momentum is the enemy** of an effective core workout.

WEEK 1	FIND YOUR CORE		
	MONDAY	**TUESDAY**	**WEDNESDAY**
Level 1	**CARDIO** HIIT Workout 1 20 min.	**SCULPT** Balance & Isometrics 1–2 sets of Exercises 1–5	**REST**
Level 2	**CARDIO** HIIT Workout 1 22 min.	**SCULPT** Balance & Isometrics 1–2 sets of Exercises 1–8	**REST**
Level 3	**CARDIO** HIIT Workout 1 28 min.	**SCULPT** Balance & Isometrics 1–2 sets of Exercises 1–10	**CARDIO** Aerobic Workout 1 25 min.

When given the option of doing 1 or 2 (or 3!) sets of an exercise, I suggest doing the lower quantity first. When you have completed all the exercises, take stock of how you feel. If you want to get a little more bang for your buck and your body says yes, then start from the beginning and do the exercises again for that second (or third) set.

THURSDAY	FRIDAY	SATURDAY	SUNDAY
SCULPT	**REST**	**SCULPT**	**REST**
Pushing & Pulling 1–2 sets of Exercises 1–5		Twisting & Bending 1–2 sets of Exercises 1–4	
CARDIO		**CARDIO**	
Aerobic Workout 1 19 min.		Low-Intensity Workout 40 min.	
SCULPT	**CARDIO**	**SCULPT**	**REST**
Pushing & Pulling 1–2 sets of Exercises 1–8	Low-Intensity Workout 45 min.	Twisting & Bending 1–2 sets of Exercises 1–6	
CARDIO			
Aerobic Workout 1 22 min.			
SCULPT	**CARDIO**	**SCULPT**	**REST**
Pushing & Pulling 1–2 sets of Exercises 1–10	Low-Intensity Workout 50 min.	Twisting & Bending 1–2 sets of Exercises 1–8	

WEEK 2

BUILD YOUR CORE

	MONDAY	TUESDAY	WEDNESDAY
Level 1	**CARDIO** HIIT Workout 2 28 min.	**SCULPT** Balance & Isometrics 1–2 sets of Exercises 6–10	**REST**
Level 2	**CARDIO** HIIT Workout 2 30 min.	**SCULPT** Balance & Isometrics 1–2 sets of Exercises 1–10	**REST**
Level 3	**CARDIO** HIIT Workout 2 36 min.	**SCULPT** Balance & Isometrics 2–3 sets of Exercises 1–10	**CARDIO** Aerobic Workout 1 25 min.

In this second week you will be asked to commit more time to both your cardio and your sculpting workouts. Make these workouts a priority—it's how you will build a kick-ass core!

THURSDAY	FRIDAY	SATURDAY	SUNDAY
SCULPT	**REST**	**SCULPT**	**REST**
Pushing & Pulling 1–2 sets of Exercises 6–10		Twisting & Bending 1–2 sets of Exercises 5–8	
CARDIO		**CARDIO**	
Aerobic Workout 1 19 min.		Low-Intensity Workout 40 min.	
SCULPT	**CARDIO**	**SCULPT**	**REST**
Pushing & Pulling 1–2 sets of Exercises 1–10	Low-Intensity Workout 45 min.	Twisting & Bending 1–2 sets of Exercises 1–8	
CARDIO			
Aerobic Workout 1 22 min.			
SCULPT	**CARDIO**	**SCULPT**	**REST**
Pushing & Pulling 2–3 sets of Exercises 1–10	Low-Intensity Workout 50 min.	Twisting & Bending 2–3 sets of Exercises 1–8	

BOOST YOUR METABOLISM

	MONDAY	TUESDAY	WEDNESDAY
Level 1	**CARDIO** HIIT Workout 3 18 min.	**SCULPT** Balance & Isometrics 1–2 sets of Exercises 1–10	**REST**
Level 2	**CARDIO** HIIT Workout 3 19 min.	**SCULPT** Balance & Isometrics 2–3 sets of Exercises 1–10	**REST**
Level 3	**CARDIO** HIIT Workout 3 22 min.	**SCULPT** Balance & Isometrics 3 sets of Exercises 1–10	**CARDIO** Aerobic Workout 1 25 min.

Week 3 is the final push before we head into a Recovery Week. Stay focused and try to maximize the quality of your movements. You've seen all the exercises at this point—make sure you aren't just phoning it in. And on those Tabata-style cardio workouts, push yourself! These are short workouts, which means the focus is on intensity.

THURSDAY	FRIDAY	SATURDAY	SUNDAY
SCULPT	**REST**	**SCULPT**	**REST**
Pushing & Pulling 1–2 sets of Exercises 1–10		Twisting & Bending 1–2 sets of Exercises 1–8	
CARDIO		**CARDIO**	
Aerobic Workout 1 19 min.		Low-Intensity Workout 40 min.	
SCULPT	**CARDIO**	**SCULPT**	**REST**
Pushing & Pulling 2–3 sets of Exercises 1–10	Low-Intensity Workout 45 min.	Twisting & Bending 2–3 sets of Exercises 1–8	
CARDIO			
Aerobic Workout 1 22 min.			
SCULPT	**CARDIO**	**SCULPT**	**REST**
Pushing & Pulling 3 sets of Exercises 1–10	Low-Intensity Workout 50 min.	Twisting & Bending 3 sets of Exercises 1–8	

WEEK 4	**RECOVER**		
	MONDAY	**TUESDAY**	**WEDNESDAY**
Level 1	**CARDIO** HIIT Workout 4 20 min.	**SCULPT** Balance & Isometrics 1 set of Exercises 1–8	**REST**
Level 2	**CARDIO** HIIT Workout 4 22 min.	**SCULPT** Balance & Isometrics 1 set of Exercises 1–10	**REST**
Level 3	**CARDIO** HIIT Workout 4 28 min.	**SCULPT** Balance & Isometrics 2 sets of Exercises 1–10	**CARDIO** Aerobic Workout 1 25 min.

You've made it through the first three weeks of building your core strength and your cardio endurance, and now your body is ready for a much-deserved recovery week. You'll notice that both the duration and the intensity of the workouts have been pulled back from Week 3. Listen to your body, and allow yourself to rest if you need it—the low-intensity cardio workouts are optional this week to allow you more time off if you need it.

THURSDAY	FRIDAY	SATURDAY	SUNDAY
SCULPT	**REST**	**SCULPT**	**REST**
Pushing & Pulling 1 set of Exercises 1–8		Twisting & Bending 1 set of Exercises 1–6	
CARDIO		**CARDIO** (optional)	
Aerobic Workout 1 19 min.		Low-Intensity Workout 40 min.	
SCULPT	**CARDIO** (optional)	**SCULPT**	**REST**
Pushing & Pulling 1 set of Exercises 1–10	Low-Intensity Workout 45 min.	Twisting & Bending 1 set of Exercises 1–8	
CARDIO			
Aerobic Workout 1 22 min.			
SCULPT	**CARDIO** (optional)	**SCULPT**	**REST**
Pushing & Pulling 2 sets of Exercises 1–10	Low-Intensity Workout 50 min.	Twisting & Bending 2 sets of Exercises 1–10	

WEEK 5	CHISEL YOUR CORE		
	MONDAY	**TUESDAY**	**WEDNESDAY**
Level 1	**CARDIO** HIIT Workout 5 25 min.	**SCULPT** Balance & Isometrics 2–3 sets of Exercises 1–10	**REST**
Level 2	**CARDIO** HIIT Workout 5 28 min.	**SCULPT** Balance & Isometrics 3 sets of Exercises 1–10	**REST**
Level 3	**CARDIO** HIIT Workout 5 37 min.	**SCULPT** Balance & Isometrics 3–4 sets of Exercises 1–10	**SCULPT** Pushing & Pulling 3–4 sets of Exercises 1–10 **CARDIO** Aerobic Workout 2 35 min.

After your Recovery week, you should feel rested and be champing at the bit to dive back into some intense workouts. In Week 5 we pump up the volume on the sculpting aspect of your schedule, meaning you'll see both more frequency and more volume in the number of sculpting workouts.

THURSDAY	FRIDAY	SATURDAY	SUNDAY
SCULPT	**SCULPT**	**CARDIO**	**REST**
Pushing & Pulling 2–3 sets of Exercises 1–10	Twisting & Bending 2–3 sets of Exercises 1–8	Low-Intensity Workout 40 min.	
CARDIO			
Aerobic Workout 2 25 min.			
SCULPT	**SCULPT**	**CARDIO**	**REST**
Pushing & Pulling 3 sets of Exercises 1–10	Twisting & Bending 3 sets of Exercises 1–8	Low-Intensity Workout 45 min.	
CARDIO			
Aerobic Workout 2 30 min.			
CARDIO	**SCULPT**	**CARDIO**	**REST**
Low-Intensity Workout 50 min.	Twisting & Bending 3–4 sets of Exercises 1–8	HIIT Workout 4 28 min.	

WEEK 6

MELT FAT

	MONDAY	TUESDAY	WEDNESDAY
Level 1	**CARDIO** HIIT Workout 6 26 min.	**SCULPT** Balance & Isometrics 2–3 sets of Exercises 1–10	**REST**
Level 2	**CARDIO** HIIT Workout 6 28 min.	**SCULPT** Balance & Isometrics 3 sets of Exercises 1–10	**REST**
Level 3	**CARDIO** HIIT Workout 6 34 min.	**SCULPT** Balance & Isometrics 3–4 sets of Exercises 1–10	**SCULPT** Pushing & Pulling 3–4 sets of Exercises 1–10 **CARDIO** Aerobic Workout 2 35 min.

You've been melting fat since you started the Core Envy program, but in this sixth week I have bumped up the caloric burn a little by adding some cardio workouts and increasing the intensity with another round of Tabata-style intervals. My challenge for you this week is to see if you can turn up the heat on the intervals. Can you push yourself a little harder during those intervals when you are at a 7–9 on the RPE scale? I know you can!

THURSDAY	FRIDAY	SATURDAY	SUNDAY
SCULPT	**SCULPT**	**CARDIO**	**REST**
Pushing & Pulling 2–3 sets of Exercises 1–10	Twisting & Bending 2–3 sets of Exercises 1–10	Low-Intensity Workout 40 min.	
CARDIO			
Aerobic Workout 2 25 min.			
SCULPT	**SCULPT**	**CARDIO**	**CARDIO** (optional)
Pushing & Pulling 3 sets of Exercises 1–10	Twisting & Bending 3 sets of Exercises 1–10	Low-Intensity Workout 45 min.	HIIT Workout 6 28 min.
CARDIO			
Aerobic Workout 2 30 min.			
CARDIO	**SCULPT**	**CARDIO**	**REST**
Low-Intensity Workout 50 min.	Twisting & Bending 3–4 sets of Exercises 1–10	HIIT Workout 6 34 min.	

WEEK 7	**SUPERCHARGE EVERYTHING**		
	MONDAY	**TUESDAY**	**WEDNESDAY**
Level 1	**CARDIO** HIIT Workout 7 19 min.	**SCULPT** Balance & Isometrics 3 sets of Exercises 1–10	**REST**
Level 2	**CARDIO** HIIT Workout 7 20 min.	**SCULPT** Balance & Isometrics 3 sets of Exercises 1–10	**REST**
Level 3	**CARDIO** HIIT Workout 7 25 min.	**SCULPT** Balance & Isometrics 3–4 sets of Exercises 1–10	**SCULPT** Pushing & Pulling 3–4 sets of Exercises 1–10 **CARDIO** Aerobic Workout 2 35 min.

This is it—the most challenging week yet! You have 6–7 days of workouts this week, so set aside the time to make this happen. You should be feeling stronger, more confident, and more familiar with the workouts. Most importantly, you should be feeling like you need a different set of workout clothes because your old ones are too big! Put your head down and focus this week; the finish line is in sight.

THURSDAY	FRIDAY	SATURDAY	SUNDAY
SCULPT	**CARDIO**	**CARDIO** (optional)	**SCULPT**
Pushing & Pulling 3 sets of Exercises 1–10	Low-Intensity Workout 40 min.	HIIT Workout 7 19 min.	Twisting & Bending 3 sets of Exercises 1–8
CARDIO			
Aerobic Workout 2 25 min.			
SCULPT	**CARDIO**	**CARDIO**	**SCULPT**
Pushing & Pulling 3 sets of Exercises 1–10	Low-Intensity Workout 45 min.	HIIT Workout 7 20 min.	Twisting & Bending 3 sets of Exercises 1–10
CARDIO			
Aerobic Workout 2 30 min.			
CARDIO	**SCULPT**	**CARDIO**	**SCULPT**
Low-Intensity Workout 50 min.	Twisting & Bending 3–4 sets of Exercises 1–10	HIIT Workout 7 25 min.	Pushing & Pulling 3 sets of Exercises 1–10

WEEK 8	**THE CHERRY ON TOP**		
	MONDAY	**TUESDAY**	**WEDNESDAY**
Level 1	**CARDIO** HIIT Workout 4 20 min.	**SCULPT** Balance & Isometrics 2 sets of Exercises 1–8	**REST**
Level 2	**CARDIO** HIIT Workout 4 22 min.	**SCULPT** Balance & Isometrics 2 sets of Exercises 1–10	**REST**
Level 3	**SCULPT** Balance & Isometrics 3 sets of Exercises 1–10	**SCULPT** Balance & Isometrics 3 sets of Exercises 1–10	**CARDIO** Aerobic Workout 1 25 min.

You've made it to the final week of your Core Envy program! You have been building core strength, burning off fat through intense cardio interval workouts, and creating a solid base of aerobic endurance thanks to the lower-intensity workouts. Weeks 5–7 saw a gradual yet substantial increase in workout volume and intensity. You have been climbing the relentless hill that is fitness, and now you have officially crested the top! In Week 8, you get to step back and enjoy the view. Look back through the workouts to appreciate how far you've come, and then look in the mirror to see how bright your fitness future is. You have achieved a stronger, sexier core!

THURSDAY	FRIDAY	SATURDAY	SUNDAY
SCULPT	**REST**	**SCULPT**	**REST**
Pushing & Pulling 2 sets of Exercises 1–8		Twisting & Bending 2 sets of Exercises 1–6	
CARDIO		**CARDIO** (optional)	
Aerobic Workout 1 19 min.		Low-Intensity Workout 40 min.	
SCULPT	**SCULPT**	**CARDIO** (optional)	**REST**
Pushing & Pulling 2 sets of Exercises 1–10	Twisting & Bending 3 sets of Exercises 1–8	Low-Intensity Workout 45 min.	
CARDIO			
Aerobic Workout 1 22 min.			
SCULPT	**CARDIO** (optional)	**SCULPT**	**REST**
Pushing & Pulling 3 sets of Exercises 1–10	Low-Intensity Workout 50 min.	Twisting & Bending 3 sets of Exercises 1–10	

TOOLS FOR TRACKING YOUR PROGRESS

You've committed to the Core Envy plan—now it's time to keep track of your results with weekly measurements and weigh-ins. Maybe it's been a while since you've stepped on the scale or taken a tape measure to your tummy, and maybe that's because you know you won't be happy with the numbers. It's one thing to have a suspicion that you've gained weight; it's another to actually have it quantified. I've gone through long periods when I refused to step on a scale or have my body fat checked, and when I finally did face the numbers, I was inevitably disappointed. *How did I let it get so out of hand? I swear I thought it was only a few pounds! How long has this been going on?*

In order to hold yourself accountable, you need to know the facts about your body. No one but you has to know the numbers, so get on that scale and grab that tape measure. Write it down, follow the Core Envy plan, and then watch those numbers go down. Your weekly check-in should be something you look forward to because it will confirm how hard you've been working.

Tips to ensure that your measurements are consistent and accurate:
- Always weigh yourself first thing in the morning with no clothes on
- If you have a scale that reads body fat, try to make sure your hydration level is consistent every time you do a reading. These scales use bioelectrical impedance to measure body fat, and your hydration level will affect the number.

Take before and after pictures in a swimsuit or workout clothes. This is for your eyes only, but you will be really glad to have that before picture. Seeing a side-by-side of how far you've come is excellent motivation to keep going!

WEEKLY CHECK-IN

MEASUREMENTS	WEEK 1	+/–	WEEK 2	+/–	WEEK 3	+/–
WAIST (smallest part of torso)						
BELLY BUTTON						
HIPS (widest part of torso)						
TOTAL						

BODY COMPOSITION	WEEK 1	+/–	WEEK 2	+/–	WEEK 3	+/–
BODY FAT %						
WEIGHT						

STARTING BODY WEIGHT:

GOAL BODY WEIGHT:

WEEK 4	+/–	WEEK 5	+/–	WEEK 6	+/–	WEEK 7	+/–	WEEK 8	+/–

WEEK 4	+/–	WEEK 5	+/–	WEEK 6	+/–	WEEK 7	+/–	WEEK 8	+/–

TOTAL
INCHES LOST:

TOTAL BODY
FAT % LOST:

CORE ENVY LOG

Date _____   Water (8 oz.) **1 2 3 4** 5 6 7 8

DIET

_____

_____

_____

_____

_____

_____

_____

_____

_____

_____

_____

_____

_____

_____

_____

_____

FOOD	PORTION	CALORIES
Vegetables	**1 2 3 4 5** 6 7	
Fruits	**1** 2 3	
Protein (including legumes)	**1 2 3 4** 5 6 7	
Fats	**1 2 3 4** 5	
Grains & Carbohydrates	**1 2 3** 4	

DAILY CALORIE GOAL _____

ACTUAL CALORIES _____

+/– _____

WORKOUT

SCULPTING

ROUTINE	SETS	EXERCISES	LEVEL

CARDIO

WORKOUT	NO.	TIME	LEVEL

BOOTY BONUS

The purpose of this section is not only to give you glutes that fire on command but also to sculpt those muscles into the roundest, firmest version of themselves!

The term "booty" refers to the gluteal muscles, which are the largest and most important muscles of the posterior side of the pelvis. If your glutes are weak, shut off, or just not firing on all cylinders, you will have a hard time both stabilizing and mobilizing your pelvis. When your pelvis isn't moving correctly, it can negatively affect all your other core exercises and can contribute to chronic low-back pain.

The exercises that follow will help activate and strengthen your glutes so that you can better utilize them during your core sculpting routines. I've included exercises that work the top, bottom, and sides of the glutes to ensure that none of the muscle fibers are ignored. Even if you don't need to work on getting your glutes to fire correctly, you might want to throw in these exercises just to get a little extra booty sculpt!

These first three exercises are all done from a quadruped position, which means on your hands and knees. Be sure to keep your hands directly below your shoulders and knees below your hips. During all three movements, work to stabilize your pelvis and low back by engaging your deep core muscles and slightly tilting your tailbone down toward the ground.

DONKEY KICKS

▸ **1 set is 15 repetitions on each leg**

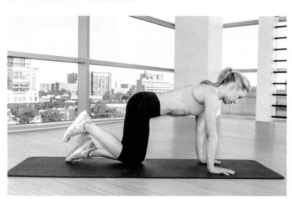 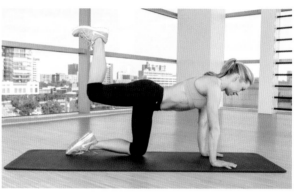

Maintain a 90-degree bend in your leg as you gently kick your foot up toward the ceiling. Squeeze your glute at the top of the movement, and don't let your low back sag or sway.

HURDLES

▸ **1 set is 15 repetitions on each leg**

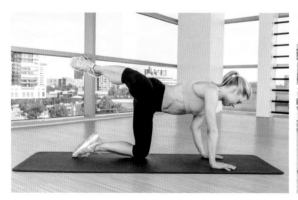 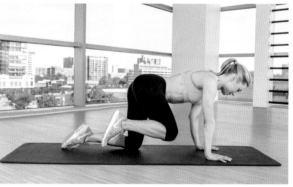

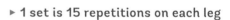

Lift your knee and sweep it back, then out, up, and around to the side as if you're trying to clear a hurdle. Try not to let your body tip to the opposite side, and keep your shoulders and pelvis parallel with the ground.

SIDE LIFTS

▶ 1 set is 15 repetitions on each leg

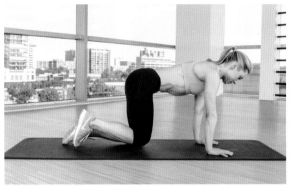 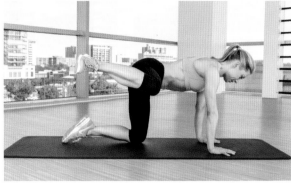

Lift your knee and take it out to the side, stopping when your knee is parallel to the ground. Try not to tip your body toward the opposite side, and keep your shoulders and pelvis parallel with the ground.

SINGLE-LEG BRIDGE

▶ 1 set is 15 repetitions on each leg

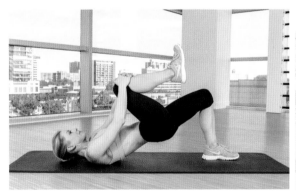 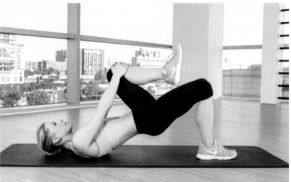

Lie on your back with your knees bent and your feet on the ground 8 to 10 inches from your glutes. Lift one leg off the floor. Pressing through the opposite heel, lift your hips as high off the ground as possible. You should feel this movement primarily in the glute of your working leg.

A few years ago I wanted to create a glute-activation exercise for a client who couldn't do any exercises that required her to bend her knees, and this is what I came up with. It has since become one of my favorite exercises, and I incorporate it into my own routines on a regular basis.

SIDE-LYING LEG LIFT WITH FORWARD KICK ▸ 1 set is 15 repetitions on each leg

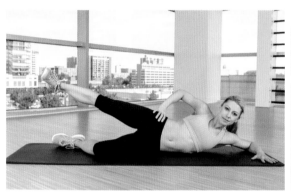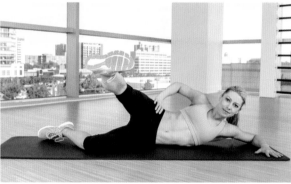

Lie on your side with your body in a straight line. Check to make sure your hips aren't pushed back behind the line of your shoulders and feet. Bend your bottom leg for support if you like. Lift your top leg approximately 2 feet and squeeze your glute. Keep your leg lifted, then move your foot forward in a kicking motion, as if you are trying to tap your toe on something 2 feet in front of your body.

NOTES

STEP 1: THE NEW RULES OF SCULPTING

1. M. S. Olson, "Analysis of Yoga, Pilates and Standing Abdominal Exercises: An Electromyographic Study," *Medicine and Science in Sports and Exercise* 44 (suppl. 5) (2010): 8–14.

2. James A Levine, "Measurement of Energy Expenditure," *Public Health Nutrition* 8 (October 2005): 1123–1132, doi:10.1079/PHN2005800.

3. S. K. Kim, H. J. Kim, K. Y. Hur, S. H. Choi, C. W. Ahn, S. K. Lim, K. R. Kim, H. C. Lee, K. B. Huh, and B. S. Cha, "Visceral Fat Thickness Measured by Ultrasonography Can Estimate Not Only Visceral Obesity but Also Risks of Cardiovascular and Metabolic Diseases," *American Journal of Clinical Nutrition* 79, number 4 (2004): 593–599.

4. PubMed Health Glossary, "Back Pain: Painful Sensation in the Back Region," http://www.ncbi.nlm.nih.gov/pubmedhealth/PMH0004668.

STEP 2: CARDIO WORKOUTS THAT MELT FAT

1. L. Kravitz, "Women and Hormones" lecture, IDEAFit World Convention (August 15, 2014); E. J. Fine and R. D. Feinman, "Thermodynamics of Weight Loss Diets," *Nutrition and Metabolism* 1, 15 (2004), doi:10.1186/1743-7075-1-15.

2. B. A. Irving, C. K. Davis, D. W. Brock, J. Y. Weltman, D. Swift, E. J. Barrett, and A. Weltman, "Effect of Exercise Training Intensity on Abdominal Visceral Fat and Body Composition," *Medicine and Science in Sports and Exercise* 40, 11 (2008): 1863–1872.

3. US Bureau of Labor Statistics, "American Time Use Survey Summary," June 18, 2014, www.bls.gov/news.release/atus.nr0.htm.

4. A. V. Chantal and L. Kravitz, "Exercise After-Burn: A Research Update," *IDEA Fitness Journal* 1, 4 (2004); D. Malatesta, C. Werlen, S. Bulfaro, X. Chenevière, and F. Borrani, "Effect of High-Intensity Interval Exercise on Lipid Oxidation During Post Exercise Recovery," *Medicine and Science in Sports and Exercise* 41, 2 (2009): 364–374.

5. American Psychological Association, "Stress in America 2013 Highlights," accessed June 9, 2015, www.apa.org/news/press/releases/stress/2013/highlights.aspx.

6. T. Coutinho, K. Goel, D. Corrêa de Sá, C. Kragelund, A. M. Kanaya, M. Zeller, J. S. Park, L. Kober, C. Torp-Pedersen, Y. Cottin, L. Lorgis, S. H. Lee, Y. J. Kim, R. Thomas, V. L. Roger, V. K. Somers, and F. Lopez-Jimenez, "Central Obesity and Survival in Subjects with Coronary Artery Disease: A Systematic Review of the Literature and Collaborative Analysis with Individual Subject Data," *Journal of the American College of Cardiology* 57, 19 (2011): 1877–1886.

7. S. Boutcher, "High-Intensity Intermittent Exercise and Fat Loss," *Journal of Obesity* (2011), doi:10.1155/2011/868305.

STEP 3: EATING FOR WEIGHT LOSS

1. J. L. Pillitteri, S. Shiffman, J. M. Rohay, A. M. Harkins, S. L. Burton, and T. A. Wadden, "Use of Dietary Supplements for Weight Loss in the United States: Results of a National Survey," *Obesity* 16 (2008): 790–796, doi: 10.1038/oby.2007.136.

2. Tim Casey, "FDA-Approved Drug and Lifestyle Changes for Obesity," First Report Managed Care, June 2014, http://www.firstreportnow.com/articles/fda-approved-drugs-and-lifestyle-changes-obesity.

3. US Department of Agriculture, "Food Availability (per Capita) Data System, Summary Findings," http://www.ers.usda.gov/data-products/food-availability-(per-capita)-data-system/summary-findings.aspx#.VErGavldWzE.

4. M. D. Mifflin, T. S. J. Sachiko, L. A. Hill, B. J. Scott, S. A. Daugherty, and O. K. Young, "A New Predictive Equation for Resting Energy Expenditure in Healthy Individuals," *American Journal of Clinical Nutrition* 51 (1990): 241–247.

5. C. K. Martin, L. K. Heilbronn, L. de Jonge, J. P. Delany, J. Volaufova, S. D. Anton, L. M. Redman, S. R. Smith, and E. Ravussin, "Effect of Calorie Restriction on Resting Metabolic Rate and Spontaneous Physical Activity," *Obesity (Silver Spring)* 15, no. 12 (December 2007): 2964–2973.

6. Martin et al., "Effect of Calorie Restriction on Resting Metabolic Rate and Spontaneous Physical Activity"; C. Weyer, R. L. Walford, I. T. Harper, M. Milner, T. MacCallum, P. A. Tataranni, and E. Ravussin, "Energy Metabolism After 2 y of Energy Restriction: The Biosphere 2 Experiment," *American Journal of Clinical Nutrition* 72, no. 4 (2000): 946–953.

7. J. DiNoia, "Defining Powerhouse Fruits and Vegetables: A Nutrient Density Approach," *Preventing Chronic Disease* 11 (2014): 130390, doi: http://dx.doi.org/10.5888/pcd11.130390; Monica H. Carlsen, Bente L. Halvorsen, Kari Holte, Siv K. Bøhn, Steinar Dragland, Laura

Sampson, Carol Willey, Haruki Senoo, Yuko Umezono, Chiho Sanada, Ingrid Barikmo, Nega Berhe, Walter C. Willett, Katherine M. Phillips, David R. Jacobs, and Rune Blomhoff, "The Total Antioxidant Content of More Than 3100 Foods, Beverages, Spices, Herbs and Supplements Used Worldwide," *Nutrition Journal* 9, no. 3 (2010), http://www.nutritionj.com/content/9/1/3, doi: 10.1186/1475-2891-9-3.

8. R. Baudrand, C. Campino, C. A. Carvajal, O. Olivieri, G. Guidi, G. Faccini, P. A. Vöhringer, J. Cerda, G. Owen, A. M. Kalergis, and C. E. Fardella, "High Sodium Intake Is Associated with Increased Glucocorticoid Production, Insulin Resistance and Metabolic Syndrome," *Clinical Endocrinology* 80 (2014): 677–684, doi:10.1111/cen.12225.

9. H. Stewart, J. Hyman, J. C. Buzby, E. Frazao, and A. Carlson, "How Much Do Fruits and Vegetables Cost?" US Department of Agriculture Economic Research Service, *Economic Information Bulletin* 71 (February 2011), http://www.ers.usda.gov/publications/eib-economic-information-bulletin/eib71.aspx.Bottom of Form.

10. B. H. Lin. and S. T. Yen, "The U.S. Grain Consumption Landscape: Who Eats Grain, in What Form, Where, and How Much?" US Department of Agriculture, Economic Research Service, ERR-50, 2007.

11. "Carbohydrates," The Nutrition Source, Harvard T. H. Chan School of Public Health, accessed August 31, 2015, http://www.hsph.harvard.edu/nutritionsource/carbohydrates.

CORE ENVY CARDIO WORKOUTS

1. S. K. Powers and E. T. Howley, *Exercise Physiology: Theory and Application to Fitness and Performance,* 6th ed. (New York: McGraw-Hill, 2007).

2. W. D. Bandy, J. M. Irion, and M. Briggler, "The Effect of Static Stretch and Dynamic Range of Motion Training on the Flexibility of the Hamstring Muscles," *Journal of Orthopaedic and Sports Physical Therapy* 27, no. 4 (1998): 295–300.

3. I. Shrier and K. Gossal, "Myths and Truths of Stretching," *The Physician and Sports Medicine* 28 (2000): 57–63.

THE CORE ENVY DIET

1. F. Batmanghelidj, *Your Body's Many Cries for Water* (Global Health Solutions, 2006); R. J. Maughan, J. B. Leiper, and S. M. Shirreffs, "Restoration of Fluid Balance After Exercise-Induced Dehydration: Effects of Food and Fluid Intake," *European Journal of Applied Physiology and Occupational Physiology* 17, no. 3–4: 317–325.

ABOUT THE AUTHOR

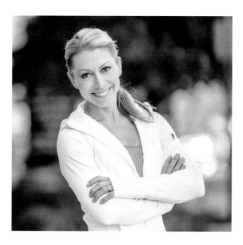

Allison Westfahl is a nationally renowned exercise physiologist, author, and fitness personality. Over the course of her highly successful career in health and fitness, Allison has worked at the nation's top health clubs, leading teams of personal trainers and shaping group fitness programs for people from all walks of life.

After growing up on a sheep farm in Kansas and graduating from Yale with a degree in classical music, Allison embarked on a personal quest for a healthier lifestyle—a quest that ultimately led her to become a personal trainer. In the years since, she has gone on to earn a master of science degree in exercise science and multiple certifications through the National Academy of Sports Medicine and endurance sports federations. Her clients range from elite cyclists, triathletes, and professional models to everyday men and women with little time for working out and lots of pounds to shed. Allison's wide range of experience and knowledge has made her passionate about creating personal training programs that deliver lasting results. Allison lives in Denver, Colorado, where she is the personal training director at Pura VidaFitness & Spa.

ABOUT THE MODELS

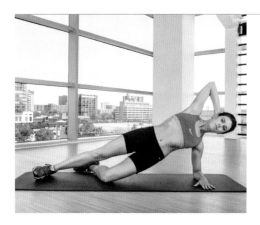

KELLY DUGAN is a fitness professional who enjoys helping people of all levels reach their fitness goals and obtain physical and mental wellness. Kelly's love for movement and physicality began with a career as a professional dancer. She has taught a variety of fitness styles and has earned multiple fitness certifications and awards. She has a degree in communications and has experience in teaching, marketing, sales, and operational management for various fitness and wellness companies.

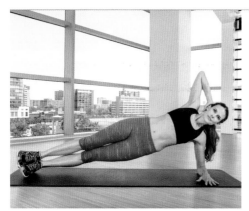

MEHGAN HEANEY-GRIER is a lifelong adventurer who specializes in pushing boundaries and thrives on personal challenges. She established the first US freedive record for both men and women in 1996, with a dive to 165 feet on a single breath of air. Mehgan is one of the original inductees into the Women Diver's Hall of Fame and holds degrees in ecology and evolutionary biology and anthropology. She heads an Ocean Ambassador Certification Program for a nonprofit organization in Colorado.

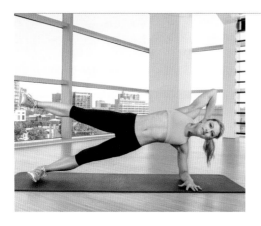

ALLISON WESTFAHL is a nationally renowned exercise physiologist, author, and fitness personality. Over the course of her highly successful career in health and fitness, Allison has worked at the nation's top health clubs, leading teams of personal trainers and shaping group fitness programs for people from all walks of life. She lives in Denver, Colorado, where she is the personal training director at Pura Vida Fitness & Spa.